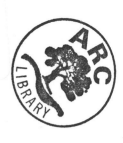
Communication Skills for Health and Social Care

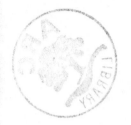

Communication Skills for Health and Social Care

Bernard Moss

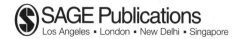

SAGE Publications
Los Angeles ▪ London ▪ New Delhi ▪ Singapore

First published 2008

 SAGE Publications Ltd
1 Oliver's Yard
55 City Road
London EC1Y 1SP

SAGE Publications Inc.
2455 Teller Road
Thousand Oaks, California 91320

SAGE Publications India Pvt Ltd
B 1/I 1 Mohan Cooperative Industrial Area
Mathura Road
New Delhi 110 044

SAGE Publications Asia-Pacific Pte Ltd
33 Pekin Street #02-01
Far East Square
Singapore 048763

Library of Congress Control Number: 2007922366

British Library Cataloguing in Publication data

A catalogue record for this book is available from the
British Library

ISBN 978-1-4129-2284-5
ISBN 978-1-4129-2285-2 (pbk)

Typeset by C&M Digitals Pvt Ltd, Chennai, India
Printed in Great Britain by The Cromwell Press Ltd, Trowbridge, Wiltshire
Printed on paper from sustainable resources

DEDICATION

This book is dedicated to Professor Christine King,
Vice Chancellor of Staffordshire University,
and to all my colleagues and social work students
past and present.

They have always drawn the best out of me
and deserve nothing less.

Contents

Foreword
by Professor Neil Thompson

I have long been fascinated by language in particular and communication in general. Throughout my professional career I have been aware of how central communication is to the effectiveness or otherwise of our endeavours – and how drastically wrong things can turn out when people do not attach sufficient significance to communication, or fail to treat it with the respect it deserves.

This book, from a highly respected educator and author, with a wealth of experience and expertise in the 'people professions', is therefore one that I very much welcome. The author's extensive knowledge base – and skill in communicating it effectively – is amply evidenced in this important work. What comes across very clearly is that here is someone who not only has an excellent grasp of the subtleties of communication as an academic discipline, but also fully understands how the theoretical underpinnings manifest themselves in the complex world of professional practice. And, as if that were not enough in itself, he also 'practises what he teaches' (there is no preaching here!), in so far as he conveys in a highly effective way his important messages about communication skills in action.

There are many books to be found on the subject of communication that are not of direct use to professional practitioners. Some are highly abstract tomes that explore certain issues in fine detail and, while there may be some important indirect, longer-term lessons to be learned from such works, their immediate value to the busy practitioner or manager is limited. Other books on communication provide a 'cookbook', how-to type slant on the subject – often risking the dangers of oversimplification that can arise from such approaches. Communication is far too complex and important a topic to be left to such a simplistic approach. There are, then, relatively few books that provide a helpful blend of theory and practice, but there is now one more to add to that short list – and what an excellent one it is too.

The use of what might be called an enhanced dictionary format (enhanced, in the sense that it is not simply a set of basic definitions, but rather is enriched by commentary, learning exercises and so on) is particularly effective in providing both an overview of the territory and helpful guidance on linking theoretical understanding to the challenges of practice. This is bound to make this a popular and successful book, and deservedly so.

High-quality professional practice is not possible without a high level of communicative effectiveness. This book will therefore be a significant contribution to developing the foundations of effective communication and thus paving the way for the high-quality practice the people we serve are entitled to.

Neil Thompson, Professor of Social Work and Well-being at Liverpool Hope University; Director, Avenue Consulting Ltd (www.avenue consulting.co.uk); and the author of *Communication and Language: A Handbook of Theory and Practice* (Palgrave Macmillan, 2003).

Acknowledgements

No book is ever written in a vacuum. My own development in communication skills is a rich tapestry of experience as a worker in a community therapy psychiatric hospital in the 1960s; training as a counsellor, and later as a family mediator and as a probation officer. For the past decade or so I have had the lead responsibility for teaching communication skills to social work students at Staffordshire University.

My reflections on communication skills have been enormously enhanced by colleagues like Pam Trevithick, whose seminal work on Social Work Skills is likely to remain the definitive core text for many years to come. But her friendship and encouragement, together with that of Julia Phillips when she was working for the Higher Education Academy Social Work and Social Policy Centre (SWAP), have been hugely influential in helping me appreciate best practice. Neil Thompson has continued to provide me with insightful wisdom through his publications and colleagueship. Mike Wolfe, formerly Chief Executive Officer of Stoke on Trent Citizens Advice Bureau and the city's first elected Mayor, has by his example taught me more about the importance of celebrating diversity and developing ways of communicating this value-base to others than he will ever realise. I am indebted to the practice wisdom of Viv Washington, who has read the manuscript and has provided me with good feedback and additional information to incorporate into the text. My insights have been deepened through a growing familiarity with how medical students are now trained in communication skills, and I hope this dictionary will be as useful to them as to other professional people-workers.

The team at Sage, especially Zoë Elliott-Fawcett and Anna Luker, have been unstinting in their encouragement to me throughout this project. They have made me feel that I have something useful to say, and it has been a privilege to work with them.

In the end, of course, the buck steps with me, and any grumbles belong in my in-tray and no-one else's.

About the Author

Bernard Moss is Professor of Social Work Education and Spirituality at Staffordshire University. He has been responsible for teaching communication skills to social work students for over a decade. His highly interactive and experiential approach to teaching has given students an opportunity to take responsibility for their own learning and development as trainee practitioners. His teaching excellence was recognised by the Higher Education Academy who in 2004 awarded him a National Teaching Fellowship.

He was part of the working group established by the Social Care Institute for Excellence to prepare a report on the literature on communication skills for social work, and has also produced a DVD on the use of large group role play in higher education.

His practice experience includes previous work as a probation officer, a family mediator and marriage counsellor, and as the founder director of the Samaritans of Wakefield and District. He has had leadership responsibilities within several faith communities including university chaplaincy. He has served on the management committees of the Stoke on Trent Citizens Advice Bureau and the North Staffordshire Community Mediation service.

His particular research and publications interests lie in the field of communication skills and in developing a wider appreciation of the contribution that an understanding of religion and spirituality can make to people-work in general, and social work in particular. He is the Director of the Centre for Spirituality and Health at Staffordshire University.

Introduction

To be human is to communicate. Whether we realise it or not, all of us all of the time are sending out messages to other people, directly or indirectly, about ourselves and others. From the way we choose to dress, to the gestures we make; from the style and choice of language we use, to the company we keep, we are all the time giving out messages to each other. Sometimes we are heard clearly; often we are misunderstood; occasionally we get it completely wrong. The complexity and fascination of communication is part of the joy of being human.

Some people choose careers and professions where communication skills are of vital importance, where getting it wrong is not an option. The seemingly endless and repetitive checking and double-checking in hospital before an operation is due in no small measure to previous poor communication within the National Health Service, resulting in the wrong leg being operated on, or the wrong person being given bad news, or confidential information being divulged to the wrong person. Communication skills are therefore at the very heart of people-work.

Aims of the book

This book is aimed at any of the helping professions for whom good communication skills are an essential part of their role. It will be of particular interest to social workers, not least because the author is deeply involved in social work education, and has many years' experience in helping students develop their communication skills for this important work. But in these days of multidisciplinary and interprofessional collaboration, it cannot be argued that there is a set of communication skills that is uniquely relevant to any one profession or discipline. Communication skills are communication skills, and it behoves anyone working with other people to take the responsibility of ensuring that these skills are developed to the highest level possible.

For this reason the admittedly somewhat inelegant term 'people-worker' has been adopted throughout. If you are involved in any way at all, professionally or in a voluntary capacity, with an agency that sets out to help people and offer support, then this book is for you. Social workers, probation officers, doctors, nurses and paramedics, teachers, police officers, youth workers, advice workers and many others who work in a wide range of 'not-for-profit' helping agencies: these colleagues are the audience that this book seeks to address. Inevitably, there will be issues which have not been covered, or which some disciplines feel should have been given a different focus. No book can be everything to all its readers. Nevertheless, the issues covered here are widely relevant, and the exercises can be used and applied by colleagues in a wide range of settings. The book is designed to stimulate and develop reflection about how to improve communication skills, and therefore also depends significantly upon the amount of energy and enthusiasm put into it by the reader to maximise its benefits.

A dictionary approach

The design of the book deserves some comment. There are many excellent books already on the market dealing with communication skills, many of them taking their readers to great depth and in great detail for particular professional groups. This book does not in any way seek to replace such volumes, or to suggest that they do not repay careful, prolonged and detailed study. They remain core texts for various disciplines. This dictionary approach, with its relevance to a variety of professional disciplines, has been adopted for the following reasons:

- It seeks to be more accessible, by drawing together the main themes for a specific topic into one discussion. In many of the other core texts on the market you often have to consult the index and consult several different pages in order to gain a full picture.
- It acts as both an introduction for a student, and as a refresher to the busy practitioner. Key issues and themes are identified to provide a good grasp and overview of the particular topic, with encouragement to deeper study by suggesting further reading and deeper reflection.
- It seeks to be especially helpful to mentors, practice teachers, supervisors and other experienced colleagues who have responsibility to help trainees and students develop their communication skills, and to develop their awareness. The exercises offered throughout the book may be used, therefore, as discussion starters or as preparatory exercises for the student to engage with, before coming to supervision.
- Its accessible, even conversational, style reflects a relationship between a tutor/supervisor/trainee and a worker or student. It seeks to talk with the reader about important themes in an encouraging and facilitative way so that they can develop their own style with confidence.

There are nevertheless some challenges to this approach. No book can ever be totally comprehensive, and inevitably there will be some readers who feel that the choice of topics has been incomplete. There is also the difficulty of avoiding unnecessary repetition. To help achieve this, some themes have been brought together into a more general discussion. The theme of a resilience and a strengths perspective, for example, are discussed under the heading of empowerment, and some of the core aspects of active listening have been explored under that heading rather than commanding an individual entry, to help achieve a coherent approach. The reader is signposted to these general discussions where necessary.

Introducing communication skills

Implicit throughout this is a comprehensive understanding of what is meant by communication skills for people-work. There are, of course, some very specific skills and techniques, such as the use of open questions and genograms, which may be seen as the people-worker's equivalent of the carpenter's ability to make mortice and tenon joints accurately. These are skills that can be identified and practised as part of the worker's communication skills toolkit, and will help them to do a better job. But communication is a far more complex phenomenon than a set of discrete skills. It is something to do with the whole person, the context in which we work, and ultimately the societal values that serve as a backdrop for the work we undertake. For this reason the entries in this book will be more than a set of definitions; they offer a far more wide-ranging and discursive approach, and will seek to track the 'ripples in the pond' that our interventions with people create. There will be some entries, therefore, which tackle a certain key theme in people-work and invite you to explore what communication skills will be important in order successfully to deal with this topic. One example of this is the entry on breaking bad news. This skill is beginning to feature strongly in the communication skills training for doctors, but anyone involved in people-work will appreciate the need to have this sensitivity developed. It is one of the distinctive features of this dictionary that such themes are given detailed treatment: it is one of many areas where practitioners feel the need for guidance and encouragement, and which are often missing from some of the standard textbooks.

There is always a danger, admittedly, of giving the impression that there is only one right way of dealing with issues. When it comes to agency guidelines and procedures, of course, practitioners need to know what to do and what course of action to follow. But with the rich tapestry of communication skills it would be far from helpful to give the suggestion that we are trying to clone people into certain behaviours. There is nothing worse than being dealt with by someone who seems to be on 'auto-pilot', and who deals with us mechanistically, without that essential spark of warm humanity. This book has a different aim altogether. It seeks to encourage the practitioner, at whatever stage they may be in their careers as people-workers, to use the entries as *pictures* and as *mirrors*. When we look at a picture we should be drawn into it, and be able to appreciate both the overall story it seeks to communicate, and also some of the fine detail that is important to the theme. It helps us learn, and to widen our appreciation. In a mirror, however, we see ourselves as we are, and this helps us appreciate ways in which we need to change and develop to improve our practice. There is a constant implicit theme throughout the book: *how will you handle issues in such a way that you can make these skills part of the 'real you' as a practitioner, so that they have an integrity and genuineness about them when you are working with someone else?* One thing you can be sure of: people will pick up very quickly whether you are conveying genuine human interest, care and concern, or whether you are simply 'going through the motions'.

It is very easy, unfortunately, to hide behind the professional practitioner role. To do your job effectively, it is important that you fulfil this professional role properly, because it highlights what you can and cannot do with and for the other person. You will want to come across as caring and friendly, but you are not there to be a friend. Your role is both time-limited and task-orientated: when the job is done, you must end the relationship and close the file. What happens afterwards is not your concern. But hiding behind the role is a different story. This is when you do the job automatically, and with little warmth; you seem 'dead behind the eyes', as if you do not really care about what you are doing; and you fall into the trap that divides the world into two groups: first, the professional, trained helpers who are the experts; they know what they are doing and are competent in their roles, and should be treated with respect and gratitude, come what may, by those who fall into the second group. These are the unfortunate ones, who are problem-laden, inadequate and unable to cope, who need help and support, and who would quickly 'go under' were it not for the service which the professionals provide. Such attitudes lead to arrogance, and undermine the essential value-base of people-work that celebrates the dignity, value and worth of each and every human being. It also denies the fact that, in their personal lives, many professional practitioners experience the full range of turmoil, failure and incompetence as does anyone else. Also, many people who go to the professionals for help and support display a far greater ability to cope and have deeper resources of resilience than is often realised. The helping relationship, therefore, that communication skills are there to facilitate, needs a measure of humility, human warmth and genuineness that respects the common humanity that we all share, and a willingness to respect and enhance the determination that other people display in tackling the problems and difficulties which beset them.

To hide behind the professional role also carries the danger of 'taking over'. However satisfying it may feel to do something for the other person – and there will be occasions when this is wholly appropriate – in the end the real 'litmus test' of our work is the extent to which the other person becomes more able to take responsibility for their own life. This is not a re-working of the tired maxim to encourage people 'to stand on their own two feet'. Society is structured in such a complex way these days that the pressures which undermine people's capacity and resilience are ever increasing. It is, however, a reflection of the value-base of people-work that respects the dignity of each individual and the strengths we all have to a greater or lesser degree. If your professional help and support can trigger a range of resources, both internal and external, to facilitate this enhanced capacity to cope, your role is validated, but to do this there has to be a valued, effective professional relationship between you.

Levels of skill

The issue of levels of skill is an important dimension to this theme. Trevithick (2005: 65) discusses the journey from basic, through intermediate, to advanced skills which social workers, and indeed all people-workers, will need to take in order to maximise their effectiveness. There are basic foundational skills, such as knowing how and when to use open and closed questions, and how to begin to forge a professional relationship, that need to be introduced to students on their education and training courses so that they can develop a basic level of confidence before they are 'let loose' on the general public. Such is the nature of people-work, however, that it is not possible to plan your progress through a set of increasingly complex stages of communication skills. A surgeon needs to do this: you would not wish to have a complete novice undertake highly complex operations: a gradual progression through the range of medical knowledge and skills is essential, with each stage needing to be effectively accomplished before taking on more advanced work. In people-work, however, it is not so straightforward. There will be types of work, of course, which demand greater experience and expertise before you can begin to undertake them: child protection, complex mental health work, specialist advice and tribunal work are examples that spring to mind. Generalist skills need to be enriched by a set of specialist knowledge and skills for such work to be undertaken successfully. But in terms of the communication skills you need to practise, there is no guarantee whatsoever that the interview that seemed on paper to be simple and straightforward will not suddenly take the worker into unchartered territory of complexity, where sensitive communication is all important. This illustrates the dilemma that supervisors and practice teachers have when selecting work for an inexperienced student: you never know what is going to happen! The approach taken in this dictionary, therefore, does not seek to give each entry a 'complexity rating': it takes for granted that the level to which you will be able to go with the person depends upon two interweaving factors: your skills at exploring, and their willingness to trust you and to go deeper.

A relatively inexperienced worker, for example, could establish a basic level of communication with the other person, and deal effectively with what sometimes is called the 'presenting problem'. This may seem straightforward enough, and may be dealt with very quickly. The real skill comes in working out whether or not the 'real' reason for the person coming to you is much deeper and more complex. To be able to explore this possibility requires a great level of sensitivity that some workers have 'in spades' from day one, while with others it takes time to develop. So the new student who is very sensitive might find that they are uncovering much deeper issues than either they or their supervisor suspected were there, *precisely because* they had the ability to explore and probe sensitively. By contrast, a worker who has not developed this capacity might find that they are getting through their case-load in double-quick time simply because they are not able to reach a deeper level.

There is no 'cut and dried' route to success in this: it almost always depends upon the indefinable quality of the 'chemistry' between worker and the other person, and the extent to which they have been able to develop a trusting relationship together. Without that, the interview is likely to remain at a relatively superficial level. But even for an excellent worker there can be pitfalls: the other person may 'put the shutters up'; factors to do with age, 'race', gender and class may prove far more influential upon the outcome than had been realised. This is what makes people-work so fascinating, rewarding, frustrating and at times bewildering, not just at the outset of your career, but all the way through. And it is for this reason that reflective practice and supervision are so essential to you throughout your career. You need always to be looking into the mirror of reflective practice to ensure that you are always giving of your best and are using your communication skills to the best effect.

Each entry therefore may be utilised by both the novice and the 'old hand': all that is needed is the professional openness and willingness to be constantly evaluating and improving your practice with the constant oscillation between getting the basics right and pushing back the boundaries of your expertise.

How best to use this book

For it to be most effective and useful, this book needs to be regarded as a working tool that can be quickly and easily accessed, as well as being an encouragement to a more in-depth reflection. However it is used, it seeks to recognise and strengthen your commitment as a practitioner to develop your communication skills, and to be a working companion in your journey towards professional excellence.

The dictionary approach enables you to go straight to the topic or theme that interests you. You will gain a brief overview by reading through the entry, but because communication skills are not to be seen in isolation from each other, you will be signposted to some related concepts dealt elsewhere in the book to broaden and deepen your knowledge and understanding.

Suggestions for further reading are provided to help you engage with topics at a greater depth. The focus in this book is on communication skills: it is not a dictionary of social work, for example, where some of the theoretical concepts would be discussed in great detail. This book is designed to help you 'operationalise' these concepts, not to provide you with a complete discussion about their complexity.

For this reason, considerable emphasis has been placed upon offering exercises throughout the book. You are strongly encouraged to undertake these as an individual task to explore and enrich your practice skills. But the book is also designed to be a resource for practice teachers, supervisors, mentors, academic teachers and trainers to use as part of their training and teaching programmes. You may well be asked therefore to study a particular entry and complete the exercise(s) relevant to that theme in preparation for your next supervision or group training event. To use the book in this way will deeply enrich your learning.

One of the distinctive features of this book is that special care has been taken to provide guidance and exercises on topics or themes which do not appear in some of the other books on the market. Breaking bad news, chairing meetings, giving presentations, exploring religious and spiritual issues as part of professional practice, are some of the topics where we feel a more detailed treatment is justified in order to maximise the usefulness of the book. For many of the topics there are parallel discussions elsewhere in the literature to which you will be signposted through further reading, enabling this book to offer a more succinct approach. Where we feel we are breaking new ground, however, we have given more space to the discussion. But this is not to suggest that word length is the only indicator of importance. Far from it!

We hope that this book will become 'well-thumbed' as a valued travelling companion in your professional practice. But the ultimate test of its usefulness will be the extent to which you commit yourself to engage with the issues we raise so that the quality of the professional relationships with the people you work with is enhanced. Travel well and practise better!

Acceptance

Acceptance is a term which has entered the common parlance of people-work, not least through the seminal works of Carl Rogers (1951), Egan (2002) and Truax and Carkhuff (1967), each of whom emphasised the importance of the personal relationship between the counsellor/worker and the 'client' in a helping relationship. They argued that it is only when a person seeking help believes that they are being accepted for who they are, without being put down or being judged, that any real progress towards change can be achieved. Upon these foundations the increasingly complex disciplines of counselling and other people-work disciplines have been built (Nelson Jones, 2006).

The roots of this approach run deep within western philosophy, and also draw particular strength from the monotheistic traditions of Christianity, Judaism and Islam, where the uniqueness of each individual and their accountability to a divine creator is a central tenet of faith. In some ways the current, postmodern fascination with spirituality is highlighting the same point, that each individual seeks their own deep sense of meaning and purpose, which deserves to be respected and valued by others.

Counselling, of course, is a discrete discipline, even though some of its skills are used by other professional groups. Counselling is not social work any more than social work is counselling. But the key tenet of acceptance, so vital to counselling, has also become part of the value base and codes of conduct not only of social work but of many other helping professions. It emphasises the importance and uniqueness of each and every person with whom the professional worker comes into contact, and their right to expect to be treated with dignity and respect.

All of this, however, is easier said than done. The big question for any worker is how to put this basic tenet of a professional value base into practice when faced with people whose behaviour is oppressive, abusing and damaging to others. Professional people-workers are called upon daily to work with people whose lifestyles blatantly contradict this value base; their victims testify to their inhumanity. The one thing that acceptance is *not*, is any sense of approval for behaviour that demeans and damages others. It is part of the responsibility of people-work professionals to protect those who are vulnerable and at risk in society, and this necessarily involves challenging those who behave oppressively towards others.

It is this tension between these two aspects of our professional value base – acceptance of each individual as unique and precious, and the protection of the vulnerable from abuse – which places this theme firmly into the arena of communication skills. It is arguably one of the most difficult skills to develop for any worker, not least because our sense of moral outrage at some people's behaviour will seep into our dealings with them, however scrupulous we are with the language we use in our interviews and discussions.

Exercise 1

To illustrate this point, imagine for a moment you have to interview someone who has committed a heinous offence against a vulnerable child or older person. The graphic details of their behaviour are outlined in your file, and you feel physically sickened that someone could do this sort of thing to another human being. Just spend a few moments quietly imagining yourself face to face with this person, and identify the feelings which are churning around inside you, and what you would like to do to them if you had them alone in a dark alley. It could, after all, have been your child, your parent or grandparent.

And now get in touch with how these feelings are manifesting themselves in how you are sitting – your facial expressions, the tenseness of your body language – how your fists so easily become clenched – and now I am supposed to accept this person? You must be joking!

If you have attempted this exercise honestly, you will be firmly in this tension-filled territory which has already been described. Your professional value base insists that you treat this individual with dignity and respect; your own humanity rebels against what they have done. It is precisely because of this tension, however, that Codes of Conduct have been drawn up to ensure that we do not allow our own feelings and (let it be said) our prejudices to get in the way of the tasks which society expects of us. The significance of the exercise you have just completed is its power to remind you how you are feeling and to make the point that, whether you like it or not, those feelings will be communicated to a greater or lesser extent to the person with whom you are seeking to work. In other words, you may be able to use all the appropriate words in your interview, but the high emotions of how you are really feeling will seep out rather like a bad smell, and will pervade and strongly influence how the other person responds. And they will respond not so much to your words, but to your non-verbal communication, which speaks to them loud and clear: you are *not* accepted.

Ways forward

The discussion so far has aimed at uncovering, as honestly as we can, the way we sometimes feel about those whom we are seeking to help. The following pointers to best practice are offered to help you begin to deal with this particularly difficult area.

Supervision and preparation

If you know you are going to have to deal with a situation that stirs up strong feelings in you, it is imperative that you prepare properly. This includes talking through with your supervisor, manager or practice teacher how you feel about this particular scenario, and being honest about your feelings. You will find, more often than not, that this discussion will help you put things into perspective and enable you to deal with the person professionally. To know that you have a safe place in which to deal with *your* feelings will enable you to provide a safe place for the other person to deal with theirs. It also opens up the possibility that your supervisor may feel that someone else should take over responsibility for this case. For example, if it has triggered off within you some deep-seated hurt which cannot be easily resolved, then it would be better for someone else to handle this particular referral.

Accept yourself

Acceptance is not just how you treat other people: it has a dimension to it that involves how you think of yourself. We all have our strengths and our weaknesses; things we are good at and things we struggle with; our personal victories and our individual wounds. The best people-workers are often those who have come to a deeper understanding and acceptance of who they are, warts and all, and who reach out to others not from a position of moral superiority, but from shared humanness. Yes, we may abhor what some people have done to hurt others, but few of us as people-workers have been able to avoid hurting people in our own relationships. The sense of our own frailty and capacity to be unloving and uncaring, however, can be channelled into a more humble approach in our work with others, and help us to realise that we all struggle with trying to make a success of our lives.

Remember to practise the basics

Your basic communication skills training is there not only for you to fall back on, but to use as an essential strategy in offering acceptance to another person. The way you introduce yourself; your tone of voice; your non-verbal communication skills; your active listening skills – all are there to be used to help put the person at their ease. Then they will begin to feel that this is a space and time for them, so that no matter what they have done, they are being listened to and accepted in a respectful and dignified manner.

Be honest

Even if the person you are working with shows no remorse for their actions, you can still legitimately raise with them how many people in society (and by implication you too) feel about how they have behaved. It is perfectly legitimate to be clear with people that their actions have damaged others and that part of your role is to help protect vulnerable people. Importantly, if they can see you as an ally to help them change their behaviour, and begin to realise that in your acceptance of them as an individual you are opening up the possibility of a changed lifestyle, you will have done them an immeasurable service. To demonstrate a belief that the person can change is perhaps one of the most important messages you can ever communicate.

Be focused

As with all people work, you will need to communicate clearly with the person you are working with why you are involved; how in partnership with them you can agree what needs to be achieved, and how this will be effected; and also what the consequences are likely to be if progress is not achieved. Accepting the *consequences* of a person's behaviour is as important as accepting the person themselves.

So far the discussion has focused on a particularly sharp set of issues that throw into high relief the tension that is inherent in this theme of acceptance. However, it is important now to widen the context in order to demonstrate its relevance to the whole range of people-work. As already noted, the communication skills aspects of the discussion arises from the value base of our work, which may be characterised by the celebration of diversity. Diversity is by definition a complex theme, but in this context it reflects the multicultural, multi-faith and multi-dimensional aspect of society. If racism, sexism, classism, disablism and homophobia are the shadows cast by oppressive world-views, then the positive aspect of it is the celebration of society where people and their chosen world-views, lifestyles and various differences are both respected and celebrated as being an enrichment of our communities. As before, it is important that you understand the implications of this value base for people-work. You need to explore your own world-view and prejudices in an honest and open way, otherwise you may jeopardise the work you seek to undertake.

Here too, however, there are points of tension for people-work practice. Not every worldview may be of equal value; some litmus test has to be applied to make judgments about whether the behaviours towards others which flow from certain world-views are deemed to be respectful or oppressive. In exploring these issues, however, the same approach as we outlined above needs to be adopted, and the same communication skills implemented, to demonstrate that acceptance is not an empty theoretical perspective, but rather a commitment and an energy which pervades all our communication with others.

Exercise 2

Choose an example of an issue that you find difficult to celebrate that reflects diversity in our complex society. Try to identify what it is about this topic which causes you disquiet. Having identified the various issues, invite your supervisor or practice teacher to help you role play a scenario where you are seeking to engage with these issues in ways that are respectful and demonstrate the value-base of acceptance. After you have done this, see if you can draw up a set of guidelines to help you develop your practice in this area.

Final thoughts

This discussion has shown how a topic like acceptance, which is fundamental to the value-base of much people-work, pervades every aspect of communication skills. It is not a neat, self-contained concept: indeed, the ease with which it can be defined belies the challenge which is inherent within it for all people-work practice. It raises for you, in all your work, both in the preparation, delivery and evaluation of your engagement with others, the powerful question of whether the person we have been working with really feels accepted as a result of your intervention. There is possibly no greater challenge.

References and Further reading

Egan, G. (2002) *The Skilled Helper: A Systematic Approach to Effective Helping.* 7th edition. Pacific Grove, CA: Brooks/Cole.

Mearns, D. and Thorne, B. (1999) *Person Centred Counselling in Action.* 2nd edition. London: Sage.

Nelson Jones, R. (2006) *Theory and Practice of Counselling and Therapy.* 4th edition. London: Sage.

Rogers, C.R. (1951) *Client Centred Therapy.* Boston, MA: Houghton Mifflin.

Trevithick, P. (2005) *Social Work Skills: A Practice Handbook.* 2nd edition. Maidenhead: Open University Press.

Truax, C.B. and Carkhuff, R.R. (1967) *Towards Effective Counselling and Psychotherapy.* Chicago, IL: Aldine.

Related concepts   Active listening; counselling; spirituality.

Active Listening

Active listening ensures that everything that a person is trying to say is fully received and understood by the listener. This includes attempting to understand not just what the person is saying with their chosen words, but what some of their underlying thoughts and feelings are, that may be conveyed as much by what they do *not* say and by their body language, as by the words they use.

The term 'active listening' is frequently used by helping professionals to underline the importance of this activity. It has several layers to it, and is not merely hearing the words which are being spoken.

Active listening is, of course, easier said than done, which is why such an emphasis is laid upon it as a core communication skill. To illustrate its complexity, try the following exercise either by yourself or with a companion.

Exercise 1

See how many different tones of voice you can use in saying the words 'I agree'. You will quickly discover that some tones of voice can contradict the words you are using, just as a very defensive body posture can have a similar effect.

This is what is sometimes called the 'music behind the words' – and it is the music which conveys the *real* meaning of what is being communicated. If the listener takes the words at face value, the real meaning will be ignored.

Of course, you may speculate why this should be so, and the reason may vary from person to person. What the exercise illustrates is that communication is a complex activity, and that if you are going to work successfully with people, your whole being must be attuned to what is being said.

It goes without saying that in any interaction with someone you are seeking to help, support or work with, you need to be clear about what you are trying to do. The listening skills that you need will vary according to the nature of the task. For example, if you are a welfare rights worker doing a benefits check for someone, you will certainly need to adopt a caring, understanding approach, but for much of the interview you will be gathering and interpreting factual information which you need to help you calculate their eligibility for particular benefits. In a similar way, a doctor or nurse may need to elicit crucial information about a patient's symptoms in order to reach an accurate diagnosis. A social worker or probation officer preparing a court report will need to elicit and interpret information about a person's behaviour. By contrast, a counsellor working with a deeply distressed person following a major loss in their life will be focusing heavily on that person's feelings, and will be exploring a very sensitive aspect of their life, which requires a different set of skills as they seek to explore and develop that person's self-awareness. Someone who is working with people whose relationships are breaking down will use the skills of trying to help each of them understand what the other is saying, and using interpretative skills to a considerable degree to help people who had become deaf to each other to begin to hear each other once more.

These examples illustrate the complexity of the listening task. One common theme, however, is the type of questions that can be used in active listening. These are commonly grouped together into two categories: open questions and closed questions.

Open questions are used when you want to help someone 'open up' about themselves, to give you some insights into how they are feeling, or to explore a situation in more depth. They do not allow a straightforward 'yes' or 'no' response, but instead invite the person to talk about the topic. For example,

- Can you tell me *how* this happened?
- *What* did your parents think about ...?
- Can tell me in your own words about ...?
- *Why* do you think that was?

Some people discourage the use of the 'why?' question as being too threatening; it can put people 'on the spot' and may make conversation more difficult, especially if it assumes that a measure of blaming is implicit or even explicit in the question (*Why* on earth did you do that?). But good communication skills are not about slavishly following a set of rules with their 'do's and don'ts': they are about developing your own style, and realising that with sensitivity and appropriate voice tones you can encourage people to open up and share their story with you.

It is your sensitivity that is all important. Not everyone will feel able to 'open up' easily and share their deep thoughts and feelings. Some need to go step by step, and to be led by the interviewer cautiously until they gain confidence to go deeper. This is why closed questions also have such an important role to play.

Closed questions invite a straightforward 'yes' or 'no' answer ('Did you hit him?'), and are necessary in gathering factual information in as straightforward a way as possible. Closed questions can give a message to the interviewee that you are in charge, know what you are doing and where you are going, and that they can put their confidence in you.

It is certainly not the case that open questions are good and closed questions bad: that is a gross caricature. Each has its part to play in a well-balanced effective interview, and it is up to you to judge which will be most appropriate and effective as the interview unfolds.

Basic skills

The complexity of active listening is well illustrated by Trevithick (2005: 123, see below for Further reading), who lists 20 basic skills involved in listening. These are:

- being as open, intuitive, empathetic and self-aware as possible
- maintaining good eye contact
- having an open and attentive body orientation of posture
- paying attention to non-verbal forms of communication and meaning
- allowing for and using silence as a form of communication
- taking up an appropriate physical distance
- picking up and following cues
- being aware of our own distracting mannerisms and behaviour
- avoiding vague, unclear and ambiguous comments
- being aware of the importance of people finding their own words in their own time
- remembering the importance of the setting and the general physical environment
- minimising the possibility of interruptions and distractions
- being sensitive to the overall mood of the interview, including what is not being communicated
- listening for the emotional content of the interview and adapting questions as appropriate
- checking out and seeking feedback wherever possible and appropriate
- being aware of the importance of timing, particularly where strong feelings are concerned
- remembering the importance of tone, particularly in relation to sensitive or painful issues
- avoiding the dangers of preconceptions, stereotyping or labelling, or making premature judgments or evaluations
- remembering to refer to theories that are illuminating and helpful, and also where appropriate, to explain, in an accessible language, theories that may aid understanding
- being as natural, spontaneous and relaxed as possible.

Put like that, listening skills may seem daunting, even impossible to get completely right. They are a challenge, and it sometimes needs a list like that to remind us that to listen actively can be one of the hardest tasks we ever undertake.

Exercise 2

By yourself, with your supervisor, or in a small group, go through the 20 skills listed above, and make sure you fully understand them. Try to think of examples to illustrate each one, and explore how you would want to put these into practice yourself.

Summarising

Summarising is a useful skill, which helps to check the pace and progress of an interview. Essentially this means taking some time out from the actual flow of the interview and trying to put into words the story so far as you perceive it. This serves several useful functions:

- it demonstrates to the interviewee that you have been listening to what they are saying and that you have grasped the main issues clearly
- it provides the interviewee with an opportunity to confirm the accuracy of your summary and (importantly) to put right any misunderstanding you may have developed
- it facilitates the process of empathy between you and the interviewee
- it provides a structured staging post in the interview to take stock and to decide how to move to the next stage
- it is also a useful technique to use when the interview 'runs into the sand' and you need to 'get unstuck'.

Obviously, in the course of an interview lasting, say, for an hour, you will not want to use this summarising technique too often: that would become tedious and mechanistic. Perhaps two of three times, including the summary you will want to offer at the very end of the interview, will normally be about right.

Paraphrasing

This is a similar skill to summarising, but it provides a narrower focus in that you can use it frequently to 'mirror' or reflect back to the interviewee a particular thought, concept or feeling they are trying to express. This skill involves putting into your own words what you think the other person is trying to express. This has several advantages:

- it enables you to show that you have been listening to the interviewee
- it provides an opportunity for the interviewee to confirm, or adjust, the feedback you have provided
- it helps to establish empathy
- it provides an opportunity for the interviewee to see themselves in the 'verbal mirror' you have provided as a stimulus for further reflection.

However, as with all 'techniques', it is important that they are used sensitively and not 'robotically': that would be extremely frustrating and counter-productive. The interviewee may end up feeling that they

18

cannot get it right because you are always changing what they have said into something 'more acceptable to you', and that is the last message you will want to convey. Use the technique if you get stuck, or feel that the other person is struggling, or you feel you need their help better to understand.

Clarifying

It will come as no surprise to you to discover that people cannot always easily put into words what they are feeling or what they need to tell you. If you need any confirmation of this statement, look no further than yourself. Think back to an occasion when you were deeply upset or distressed and had to talk to someone. The chances are that all your usual confidence and articulacy somehow drained away, and you were left groping for the words that could express how you felt.

There will be occasions in an interview, therefore, where it is likely that you will not understand what is being said, for whatever reason. The skills of clarifying are important, because you do not want to get to the end of a long complex interview and still feel in the dark about some key issues and facts.

The important thing to remember here is that the interviewee will be doing their very best to communicate clearly, often under difficult circumstances. So you do not want to give out a message that they are 'making a hash' of it. Instead, it is important that you take responsibility for not fully understanding, and ask them to help you to gain the fuller picture. As is so often the case in interviewing, you need to find a form of words that feels right to you: there is no magic mantra which will always work. But something like the following may be helpful to start you off in your search for your own best approach:

> J, you have given me a very clear picture of how upset all this has made you feel. I wonder if you can help me with some of the details which I'm afraid I have not been able to sort out in my own mind yet.

> Gosh J, this is a very difficult situation – no wonder you feel so ...; I wonder if you could help me understand a bit better about 'X'.

> J, this is like a jigsaw – you have explained very clearly about 'x' and 'y', but I need your help please to understand about 'z' and how this fits into the overall picture.

> J, I wonder if it would help if we put some of the things you have told me up here on the flip chart – it would certainly help me get a better picture.

You might also find that the use of a genogram or an ecomap is a good way of clarifying the picture.

Further issues

There are additional complexities to be taken into account. They may be stated briefly but each of these issues deserves detailed consideration and reflection. The issues are gender, age, race and disability.

Gender The impact of gender must not be overlooked. For some people, and within certain cultures, it is of great importance that women have the opportunity to talk with a female worker, just as in medical matters many women prefer to have a female GP. Similarly, in some cultures, a man would want to be able to talk things over with a male worker. But even if there are not cultural imperatives to consider, this dimension will always be present, and it is important that as a worker you think about what impact this will have upon each professional encounter you experience. There will be occasions when you need to raise this issue specifically with the other person so that it can be appropriately addressed and not fester.

Age There is no denying that ageism can sometimes undermine a relationship you are trying to develop. For example, a very young worker at the outset of their career may meet with a much older person who may be tempted to disregard their expertise and potential effectiveness simply on the grounds of age and assumed inexperience. By contrast, a much older worker, when trying to work with a younger person, may find that they represent a parent figure so strongly that the young person 'puts up the shutters' and refuses to have anything to do with them. There are no easy ways round this. Sometimes it is a question of how 'cases' are allocated within an agency. What is important, however, is that you will need to raise these issues directly and try to talk about the 'blocks' that are being put up, in the hope that by airing them they can gradually be removed, and a trusting relationship established. That will be a challenge to your communication skills admittedly, but until the 'block' is identified it will not be possible to move forward.

Race One of the tenets of anti-racist practice is that, ideally, people should be able to have a worker from a similar ethnic background to themselves, to help ensure that they are fully 'heard' and that a fully sensitive assessment is made. This involves being aware that for many black and minority ethnic people to go to a predominantly white agency carries the risk of a continuation of racist attitudes and behaviours. However welcoming an agency may try to be with multicultural welcome posters on display, the reality of only being able to offer a white worker can be worrying for a member of a minority ethnic group in this country. It is important to state clearly that this fear or misgiving will have been based on previous experiences of living in a racist community, so the onus must be upon a white worker to acknowledge these issues in a sensitive way, and to check out how best to proceed. There are many examples where this 'checking out' has led to a reduction in mistrust and misgivings, and a good working relationship has subsequently been established with good outcomes. The crucial thing, however, is for white workers to be honest about the issues; to acknowledge that it can be difficult for a predominantly white agency to provide sensitive and appropriate services; and to take the initiative in talking about these issues at the first meeting.

It must also be said, however, that workers from minority ethnic groups can sometimes experience racist behaviour from white people seeking to use the service, and who express resentment that they cannot be seen by a white worker. This calls for strong anti-discriminatory policies by the agency to support all their staff and to make it clear that all members of staff are committed to delivering the best possible service to everyone who needs it. But discriminatory behaviour towards staff should not be tolerated.

Disability   All organisations need to ensure that their services are disability-friendly. This means that those who seek to use the services of the agency must be able fully to access them, and that the agency must also be able to be a disability-friendly employer. There are of course some particular challenges, for both staff and the users of the service, when working with people who are Deaf or hard of hearing; people who have communication difficulties, or lack of vision. It is important that due consideration is given to these issues so that people are not marginalised and excluded from services.

Exercise 3

Spend some time thinking through by yourself, with your supervisor, or with a group of colleagues, what the challenges are for communication skills with the four issues outlined above for your particular service or agency.

Language and dialect   One further set of issues deserves adding to the list of complexities for active listening skills. It is best practice that people who wish to access services should be able to do so in their language of choice. This will mean that on occasion you will need to negotiate for a skilled professional interpreter to be present for your interviews, so that information can be accurately exchanged. Your agency should be able to access interpreter services in your area. This includes British Sign Language for people who are Deaf. Somewhat more complicated, however, is the issue of dialects, especially if you are new to an area and are unfamiliar both with the music of the local dialect and some of the words and phrases which for local people enrich their sense of identity, but which can significantly disempower a worker seeking accurately to communicate with them. There is no substitute for seeking out some local people who would be willing to spend some time with you, helping you to become attuned to the dialect and giving you a glossary of common terms which are used. But until you are comfortable you will need to develop the skill of asking sensitively for explanations and translations, in a way which makes it clear that it is you who are on the learning curve: it is not the other person's fault!

Exercise 4

What are the issues around language and dialect in your area? How are you dealing with these?

Final thoughts

Active listening skills are complex, but they are the fundamental bedrock of good practice. They cannot be taken for granted. They need to be worked at, and as we have seen, some of the issues you will need to explore and deal with may be particularly challenging. But without good listening skills, your people-work career will never get past first base.

Further reading

Trevithick, P. (2005) *Social Work Skills: A Practice Handbook*. 2nd edition. Maidenhead: Open University Press.
Thompson, N. (2002) *People Skills*. 2nd edition. Basingstoke: Palgrave Macmillan.
Thompson, N. (2003) *Communication and Language: A Handbook of Theory and Practice*. Basingstoke: Palgrave Macmillan.

Related concepts   Acceptance; ecomaps; empathy; genograms; getting unstuck; interpreters.

Adult Learning

(*see* reflective practice)

Advising

Across the wide spectrum of people-work, advice giving – or advising – receives frequent mention, either in terms of what the organisation offers to those who use its services, or what is definitely not on offer. In counselling, for example, and in organisations such as the Samaritans, there is a strong ethos against giving advice. For this range of people-work, giving advice can be counter-productive: it smacks of telling people what to do; of making people's decisions for them, or pointing them in certain directions, with the implicit assumption that the professional knows best. In counselling, therefore, the worker's role is to help the person being counselled to think through and decide the course of action that they feel is best for them, and for which they, and they alone, can take responsibility. It would be arrogant, dangerous even, for someone else to take that responsibility away from the individual. It may well be appropriate to help someone understand the likely consequences of a certain course of action, but ultimately the decision has to lie with them.

By contrast, there are other organisations and professional people-workers where advice giving is their raison d'être. If we need to understand some legal, technical, medical or financial matters, we naturally go to those people who have accredited expertise and who can explain things to us, and advise us accordingly. Any decisions remain ours to take, but they will be taken in the light of professional advice we have received from appropriate experts.

In between are a range of people-workers, such as social workers, youth and community workers and probation officers, whose role may include an advice-giving element (for example, welfare benefits advice) alongside a combination of care and control responsibilities. Decisions about people's lives may sometimes have to be taken against their express wishes, in order either to safeguard themselves or to protect vulnerable people and children in their care. In such scenarios, a social worker may well advise someone about their rights, but will still take their child into care if that is deemed necessary.

Alongside all of this is the ever increasing independent advice sector known as Advice UK (www.adviceuk.org.uk) and the Citizens Advice network of bureaux, which exists to give to anyone who needs it free, confidential and impartial advice across a wide range of issues, including welfare benefits, debt, housing, immigration and employment. Trained volunteers spearhead this service, but professionally trained workers are also involved, sometimes as a result of commissioning by the Legal Services Commission (www.legalservices. gov.uk). Welfare rights and other forms of advice are also commonly made available in social services departments and a range of healthcare settings.

This brief overview indicates the complexity of advice and advice-giving services, and highlights the difficulty in providing a succinct definition of what advice is. In their advice work monograph, Robson and Savage (forthcoming) suggest that,

> Advice work can best be described in terms of an alloy, a composite of a range of functions which when welded together form the basis of what is generally described as 'advice work'.

As far as the communication skills needed for advice work are concerned, it is important to recognise that the government has made strenuous efforts in recent years to establish standards for advice giving which, although targeted primarily at legal advice work, also provide a quality framework for all advice-giving organisations. The Community Legal Service Quality Mark (April 2000) (www.legalservices.gov.uk) seeks to regularise processes and procedures, while the National Occupational Standards (NOS) for Legal Advice (April 2000) (www.nos4advice.org.uk) provides some benchmarks for the functions and activities performed by advisers, with 30 generic skills-based standards as well as 34 knowledge-based standards (Robson and Savage, forthcoming).

Robson and Savage outline the key communication skills in advice work as follows:

> Non-verbal skills; active listening, questioning, summarising, paraphrasing, presenting/explaining/interpreting information; checking/clarifying understanding; using the telephone; written skills; letter writing; form filling, presenting information; negotiation (persuading and influencing) and advocacy (representation-verbal presentation skills).

Exercise 1

Choose an example of some work you have done which involved giving advice to someone. Explore the work you did by itemising the exact nature of what was being asked of you, and the response you gave. Now look up the National Standards for Advice (www.nos4advice. org.uk) and use these as a checklist for the work you have chosen to analyse. How do these NOS help you understand your role as an advice-giver, and how might these NOS have helped you deal differently with this person?

Final thoughts

It will be clear from this discussion that advice giving uses the full range of communication skills that many other professional helpers utilise, and that these are essential in order to maintain the high standards of the agencies involved.

Further reading

Finch, E. and Fanfinski, S. (2007) *Legal Skills.* Oxford: Oxford University Press.

Robson, H., Savage, M. et al. (forthcoming) *Defining Advice: Advice Work Monograph.* Staffordshire University.

Taylor, M. (2005) *Negotiation.* Inns of Court School of Law. Oxford: Oxford University Press.

Wolfe, M. and Ivison, J. (2004) *Debt Advice Handbook.* 4th edition London: CPAG.

Related concepts   Active listening; advocacy; establishing a professional relationship.

Advocacy

The dictionary definitions of advocacy describe the role as being 'one who pleads the case of another'; in other words, to defend, support and to argue positively on behalf of someone else (Chambers Twentieth Century Dictionary). This seemingly straightforward definition does not, however, reflect the complexity of advocacy as an activity which is practised by a range of people-workers and others. For example:

- In court a solicitor or barrister will advocate on your behalf by providing detailed and sometimes legally complex information and opinion to the magistrate or judge.
- Social workers and health workers will from time to time speak up on behalf of their service user, client or patient to support their claim for a particular welfare benefit or a claim to housing.
- A social worker or youth worker may well speak up for a young person who is finding it difficult to find employment, and help them to obtain a job interview.
- A Citizens Advice Bureau adviser will represent you and speak on your behalf at a tribunal.
- Someone involved in Citizen Advocacy may simply act as a befriender or encourager to someone who lacks confidence, perhaps because of emotional difficulties, medical problems or a learning difficulty, and will help them put forward their views.
- A group of people may get together as a self-advocacy group or organisation to help further their cause or to seek an improvement in their circumstances. This is sometimes referred to as Peer Advocacy.

This spectrum – from the 'hard end' of legal advocacy to the 'softer' informal style – involves to a degree all the skills needed for effective advocacy, even though some forms of advocacy may require specific training and experience (for example, legal advocacy and Citizens Advice Bureau work).

Exercise 1

Spend a few moments thinking about a situation where you have been involved in an advocacy role. Note the main issues involved – what were you called to do? Were there any difficulties or dilemmas for you? Where do you think the real power lay? What was the outcome of the advocacy? How did it make you feel?

The issues you have identified in this exercise will form a useful background to this discussion, and we invite you to refer back to your experience when reflecting on the issues being raised.

The first point to stress is the importance of being very clear in your own mind what the issues are. Without such clarity you could end up in a complicated and confused situation. You also need to be clear, when considering your role, exactly what it is you are being asked to do. Will you be speaking up on behalf of the person, representing their views and needs, and being their sole mouth-piece? Or will your role be to facilitate and encourage *them* to do the talking, with you remaining in the background as a friendly support? In other words, will you be working for them, or will they be working for themselves, but with your support?

Ethical considerations

We have made it clear in the introduction that any discussion about communication skills has to include an ethical dimension. Skills are not used in a moral vacuum, but reflect the values of the person using them. It is important therefore in advocacy work to ensure that the formal communication skills are used within the basic principles of this type of work.

Bateman (1995: 26–41) highlights six main principles for what he describes as 'principled advocacy' which, although drawn from a legal context and using the legal language of 'clients', are relevant across a wider range of advocacy work. These principles are:

- act in the client's best interests
- act in accordance with the client's wishes and instructions
- keep the client properly informed
- carry out instructions with diligence and competence
- act impartially and offer frank, independent advice
- the advocate should maintain the rules of confidentiality.

Each of these principles merits detailed discussion and reflection, and you may find it useful to explore their implications for the situation you analysed in Exercise 1.

To be an effective advocate you will need the full range of interpersonal communication skills, linked with a capacity to grasp at times complex issues and to formulate and propose solutions. You will need:

- To have the self-confidence to stand up for vulnerable people, and to be willing to stand your ground when challenging organisational bureaucracy.

- To be able to interpret complex issues and to help the person you are representing, or whom you are supporting, to understand what is going on, and to be able to produce an effective response.
- Sometimes to accept that you feel inadequate and powerless against the big battalions, but if you are well prepared and know that you have a strong case to present, then you need to have the courage 'to stick with it'. At such times your own value-base, and your commitment to social justice, will stand you in good stead.

There is a further complex issue that surrounds advocacy, and that concerns power. Everything in the last paragraph is important for the advocate, but it must be tempered with the realisation that power is very tempting, and seductively 'powerful'. It gives us a good feeling to be powerful; it appeals to our sense of achievement and doing a good job, and there is a real 'buzz' when we win a tribunal or gain some advantage for a vulnerable person or family. But there is a risk here: we can too often take over, and by the effective use of our skills we can disempower those with whom we work. Sometimes it is far more important to spend time empowering others to 'fight their own corner' rather than to rely on the professional 'expert'. It can also be far more rewarding for us to take pride in watching them succeed, however falteringly at first, in presenting their own case. It is part of our skill, of course, to recognise where this is an appropriate strategy.

Exercise 2

Look at a recent copy of *Community Care* or a similar magazine such as *One in Seven* and see how many situations you can identify which warrant an advocacy approach. What do you think would be the most effective approach to use, and why?

Final thoughts

Effective advocacy is perhaps one of the most difficult skills to develop, but arguably one of the most rewarding in that you are playing a key role not only in helping someone to be fully valued, respected and at times 'rewarded', but also in helping them to gain confidence and to develop assertiveness on their journey towards greater independence.

References and Further reading

Bateman, N. (1995) *Advocacy Skills: A Handbook for Human Service Professionals*. Aldershot: Arena.

Boon, A. (1999) *Advocacy*. 2nd edition. Cavendish Legal Skills series. London: Cavendish Publishing Ltd.

Trevithick, P. (2005) *Social Work Skills: A Practice Handbook*. 2nd edition. Maidenhead. Open University Press. (pp. 232–235)

Robson, H. and Savage, M. (2007) *Defining Advice*: *Advice Work Monograph*. Stoke on Trent: Staffordshire University (unpublished).

Related concepts Advising; partnership working; empowerment, resilience and a strengths perspective.

Anti-discriminatory Practice

In all aspects of people-work, anti-discriminatory practice (ADP) not only forms part of the core value-base; it also comprises a set of communication skills through which that value-base is put into practice. ADP facilitates the celebration of diversity in our complex, multi-layered, multicultural and multi-faith society. ADP skills, therefore, involve cultivating an awareness of how prejudice and oppression operate at various levels in society to certain people's disadvantage, and then actively working to restore the balance so that people get a better opportunity to live full and creative lives.

In many ways it has been social work that has led the way in our understanding of how ADP is at the heart of best practice, but the basic principles can apply to all aspects of people-work, particularly in the field of health and social care. One author who has shaped our understanding of ADP is Thompson, whose seminal writing in this area has been hugely influential (Thompson, 2006, for example). Thompson stresses that best practice must take into account three interlocking dimensions to the ways in which prejudice and oppression can operate:

the personal (P), the cultural (C) and the structural (S). This theoretical and conceptual framework argues against too simplistic an understanding of the issues surrounding discrimination. An individual white worker, for example, may strenuously uphold a commitment to anti-racist practice, and this commitment may permeate that worker's individual personal dealings with members of the black community. But this does not alter the fact that at wider levels, in various cultural aspects and in how society is structured, racism is still a powerful, negative force which diminishes black people's life-chances. It must be dealt with.

Exercise 1

It is important to take time fully to explore the concept of ADP, and the contribution which the PCS analysis makes to our understanding. Obtain a copy of Thompson's book *Anti-discriminatory Practice* (4th edition), and read carefully the first two chapters, where the main themes are explored and discussed. This will give you a firm base upon which to develop your ADP skills.

This PCS analysis provides the framework for exploring the range of skills that are needed to put it into effective practice. Thompson puts the practice issues succinctly when he states that:

There is no middle ground; intervention either adds to oppression (or at least condones it) or goes some small way towards easing or breaking such oppressions. In this respect, the political slogan, 'If you are not part of the solution you must be part of the problem', is particularly accurate. An awareness of the sociopolitical context is necessary in order to prevent becoming (or remaining) part of the problem. (Op cit.: 15)

This suggests a set of basic questions that you can ask about your professional practice with a service user, enquirer, or client. These questions include:

- What are the issues which rightly remain in the domain of this person as an individual over which a measure of control or influence can be exerted by them, with or without your help?
- To what extent are this person's problems and difficulties due to wider influences, from family, peer group or other cultural groupings?

- How far are this person's difficulties and problems a result of structural issues and influences? Is this individual being blamed or 'pathologised' as a result of these influences?
- What course(s) of action are open to me, and to both of us working in partnership, to tackle some of the wider issues we have identified?

Exercise 2

Think about some of the people you have worked with, or are currently working with. You will probably have a clear idea about the person's difficulties and problems at the personal individual level (P). Now spend some time reflecting on wider influences at the cultural (C) and structural levels (S), and explore ways in which you think these wider issues might be addressed. Discuss this with your practice teacher or supervisor.

Because ADP is best practice and must therefore permeate all aspects of people-work, it is difficult to know what issues not to include in this brief introductory discussion. Certainly key themes such as empowerment, acceptance and partnership working are all central, as is the use of good active listening skills. The following skills, however, deserve particular mention.

Non-verbal communication In the discussion on non-verbal communication, the point is emphasised that we convey a huge amount of information to another person non-verbally, including our attitude towards them. In a variety of subtle ways we can convey dislike, disapproval, hostility even, which will be picked up by the other person. They will be made to feel that, for whatever reason, we are being discriminatory, and this may well reinforce other similar messages which they have received from society in general. It is imperative, therefore, that from the very first moment of meeting, we convey a genuine warmth and welcome.

Cultural sensitivity The service we offer to people needs to be accessible to all members of the community. This is not always easy, of course. Many organisations report that members of minority ethnic communities, or Deaf people, for example, do not make use of their services. They can feel alienated and that the service is not for them, in spite of the rhetoric and the multi-lingual notices of welcome. On occasion this is a profoundly accurate perception, and organisations need to look long and hard at ways in which they can improve their inclusivity and the 'community ownership' of their service.

On a one-to-one basis, however, cultural sensitivity is an extremely important aspect of ADP. How you greet people; how you handle gender issues; how you acknowledge the differences between you; whether you offer the services of someone who can enable people to use their first language in the interview – these and many other issues are all significant for ADP. No book or training notes can ever cover all aspects of this, of course. It is, however, incumbent upon you to become familiar with the cultural issues of the area in which you work, and to ensure that you make a serious attempt to put this into practice.

Personal awareness   Personal awareness is an important aspect of all people-work. It includes our understanding of why we undertake this type of work; what the rewards are and what needs within us are being met by doing it. It also involves being aware of key aspects about ourselves: our age; 'race'; gender; class; sexuality; disability; religious background. All of these components make us who we are, and are part of the package of what we communicate to people directly or indirectly when we work with them. Sometimes who we are – our background – will make it easier to work with some people. A shy Asian woman coming into an agency may be hugely relieved to be met by a female Asian worker of a similar age: an immediate rapport may be that much easier to establish. By contrast, a young person may feel that the older worker who is trying to relate to them cannot possibly understand 'where they are coming from', and represent unwelcome parental and authority figures. The crucial thing to bear in mind is for the worker to be aware of some of these potential advantages and disadvantages, and to be open and honest about them. Sometimes just the act of putting these hesitations into words, and trying to empathise with the other person about these issues, is enough to begin to break down potential barriers to communication.

Being open and critical about our own practice   The concept of being a reflective practitioner is now well established in people-work, thanks in no small measure to the seminal work of Schon (1983; 1987). This covers a range of issues, including self-awareness and the impact we have upon the people with whom we seek to work. The key point to make here, however, is that the skills of being a reflective practitioner need constantly to be honed and evaluated: there is no guarantee we will get it right. In fact, there is more than an even chance we will get it wrong, to some extent at least. Human diversity and complexity makes this almost inevitable. Therefore we need to have good systems in place to review what we do and how we do it, and to evaluate the impact and outcomes of our work. Supervision is one obvious mechanism for this, particularly if you are still in training, when your practice teacher or supervisor should regularly raise issues about ADP with you.

It is also good practice to devise ways of seeking feedback from the service users themselves: they, after all, are the experts in their lives and how you have interacted with them. This is not always straightforward however. Sometimes people tell you what they think you are hoping to hear! Sometimes their feedback depends upon the extent to which you have been able to deliver what they were hoping to receive. In an era when resources are being cut back, a disappointed service user may reflect that disappointment in the feedback, rather than offer a dispassionate objective evaluation of your practice. But this should not deter you from seeking feedback. Some agencies have a post-event feedback sheet which they send out; or they make a phone call to elicit comments. It is often helpful for a third party to seek this information, such as a supervisor or practice teacher. There is no one single, right or best way of seeking this feedback: what is important, however, is that you make it part of your practice to seek it out, and to reflect carefully on what is being said.

Cultivating the wider picture   An awareness of the PCS analysis should mean that with every piece of work you undertake with someone, these wider perspectives are consciously brought into play. In the discussion about assessment, the concept of 'helicopter vision' is used precisely to capture the importance of this holistic approach. This ensures that you take into account wider pressures and influences which may have shaped the person's attitudes and behaviour, and also that you draw back from a facile pathologising of a person's problems. Although each and every one of us has a measure of personal responsibility for the worldview we have chosen to make sense of our lives and the actions we take, it is often the case that wider pressures make certain undesirable outcomes inevitable. In such cases (spiralling debt is a classic example), a response of blaming the individual can be hugely discriminatory, whereas a holistic approach informed by the PCS analysis can be liberating and emancipatory.

Acknowledging and using our shared humanity   This is a skill that is rarely recognised and acknowledged in professional literature, but in many ways it is the supreme communication skill in ADP. It is far too easy to adopt the 'I'm the confident professional, the expert, and I know what is best for you' approach, while underneath we are often hurt, confused and unsure about ourselves at the person-level and in our own relationships. If we are honest, we are as susceptible to making a mess of things as anyone else, and often do just that. There is a skill, of course, in not allowing our own 'stuff' get in the way of our professional relationships. To burden someone else with our problems, or to suggest in some superficial way that to share something of our own hurts will prove therapeutic to the other person, is widely recognised as being unhelpful, even dangerous. Our hurts may inform and even underpin our capacity to empathise with the other person, but they must stay firmly in the background.

There is nevertheless a subtle communication skill at work here. If we recognise and acknowledge our shared humanity with those we become involved with professionally, it will not only save us from the professional arrogance that distances ourselves from people; more importantly, it will communicate itself to the other person that we too are human, vulnerable, and at times hurting, as well as being resilient, capable and open-hearted. If there is a tacit recognition that such capacities are open to us all, then we may be far more effective as 'wounded helpers' (Nouwen, 1999) than we realise.

Exercise 3

It is difficult sometimes to acknowledge our own hurts, but we owe it to ourselves, our commitment to best ADP, and to those who come to us for help, to be aware of situations where we begin to feel uncomfortable in our dealings with others because the issues are too close for comfort. Spend some time reflecting on your own life and areas where your own hurts may possibly get in the way of your dealings with others. Have you noticed a tendency to shy away from similar 'problem areas' in others, or to be tempted to 'share your own problems with them'? In what ways do you think you can learn how to acknowledge a shared humanity while still maintaining professional boundaries?

Final thoughts

There has been a fascinating development to the discussion of ADP in the contemporary debate about spirituality. This is seen to be a far-reaching concept that includes religion but also has far wider ramifications. Spirituality seeks to raise issues about meaning and purpose in people's lives, and to ask questions about the world-view which people choose, consciously or unconsciously, in order to make sense of the world and their place within it. Some also argue for a social justice dimension to spirituality. Moss (2005: 71), for example, argues that this concept of a person's world-view, and the impact that a person's spirituality (S) has upon their lives in both positive and negative ways, is an important component of each level of the PCS analysis, and may even warrant its own additional 'category' (S for Spiritual), thereby developing it into a PCSS analysis.

References and Further reading

Moss, B. (2005) *Religion and Spirituality*. Lyme Regis: Russell House Publishing.

Nouwen, H. (1999) *The Wounded Healer: In Our Woundedness We Can Become a Source of Life for Others*. London: Darton, Longman and Todd.

Schon, D. (1983) *The Reflective Practitioner*. London: Temple Smith.

Schon, D. (1987) *Educating the Reflective Practitioners*. San Francisco, CA: Jossey Bass.

Thompson, N. (2006) *Anti-Discriminatory Practice* 4th edition. Basingstoke: Palgrave Macmillan.

Thompson, N. (2003) *Communication and Language – A Handbook of Theory and Practice*. Basingstoke, Palgrave Macmillan.

Trevithick, P. (2005) *Social Work Skills: A Practice Handbook*. Maidenhead, Open University Press. (pp. 215–6 and *passim*)

Related concepts   Acceptance; active listening; assessment; empathy; empowerment; feedback; non-verbal communication; partnership working; spirituality.

Assessment

There can hardly be any aspect of people-work that does not involve the skill of assessment in one form or another. From the doctor making a complex diagnosis, to the solicitor trying to obtain a true picture of what happened when an offence took place; from the social worker having to make decisions about whether a child or a vulnerable adult needs care and protection, to a manager of a care home having to decide whether someone is able to go into the town safely if unaccompanied: these are some examples to illustrate the ways in which we can be called on to make assessments and judgments about other people.

At the less formal end of the spectrum, we all use some of these skills in our everyday life, when we make provisional assessments about another person's trustworthiness, for example. Of course, we some-times get it wrong: we allow our prejudices and assumptions to cloud our judgment about the other person, but nevertheless we use assess-ment skills every day of our lives.

Within the professional context of people-work, however, assessment skills are of fundamental importance as they will frequently determine what level of service, if any, a person is entitled to receive. The evalu-ation of risk features strongly in this: we may be called upon to assess whether a person constitutes a risk to themselves or to others. Then we need to devise responses that are not authoritarian or oppressive, but which work in partnership with the person involved. Taking an older person out of their home environment and placing them into residen-tial care for their own protection when their various faculties are begin-ning to fail may be a wholly inappropriate response, for example. It may be far better to consider offering some support in their own home to enable them to stay in familiar surroundings with their pride intact.

The professional literature provides detailed discussions on assess-ment, especially for social work, and it is not appropriate to summarise all the main issues here. It is useful, however, to draw attention to the very clear definition of assessment provided by Coulshed and Orme (1998: 21) who maintain that:

> Assessment is an ongoing process, in which the client participates, whose purpose is to understand people in relation to their environment; it is a basis for planning what needs to be done to maintain, improve or bring about change in the person, the environment, or both.

In identifying the communication skills inherent in all good assessment work, there are three skills-sets which are of crucial importance that may be summed up as (1) helicopter vision; (2) partnership working; and (3) passing the 'abducted by aliens' test.

Helicopter vision

Social work is not alone in its commitment to holistic assessment: care for the whole person is a concept which pervades much nursing and medical practice, for example. The real challenge which social work seeks to meet, however, is to take this holistic approach absolutely seri-ously, and to devise responses to individual problems and situations that take into account the wider contexts in which people live their lives. This is what Thompson (2005: 64) means by 'helicopter vision': it is the determination to gain as detailed and as comprehensive an overview as possible of the 'person in context'. This means, therefore, that we do not just focus on the physical, emotional, psychological and spiritual aspects of a person's life, but also explore the social, cultural and societal dimensions which may impact upon their immediate difficulties. For example, the impact of poverty, racism, disablism, the 'debt culture', or homophobia on a person's life may be of huge importance, and any solution that does not take into account these factors is bound to be short-lived.

In terms of communication skills, therefore, an effective assessment will attempt to explore these wider issues and their impact upon the person. This approach also counteracts the pathologising tendency among some welfare professionals to assume that a person's problems are all their fault, whereas the reality is often that the person has been struggling valiantly against massive societal pressures. To be able to appreciate these wider dimensions to a person's difficulties can be a significant aspect of empathic attunement, and can help them re-direct their energies towards structural, as well as individual solutions.

Exercise 1

Choose a scenario you have been involved with, and practise using the helicopter vision. What are the wider societal and cultural factors that may exacerbate this person's difficulties? How does an appreciation of these wider issues help you come to a richer assessment of what this person really needs?

Partnership working

This is a theme that pervades all social work practice, but is important in many other aspects of people-work. For it to be more than a 'practice mantra', however, it requires you to develop and practise a range of communication skills which at all levels give the clear signal to the other person that partnership working really is 'the name of the game'.

It is temptingly easy for professional workers not only to feel that 'they know best', but also to convey this to the person they are working with. From this there flows a subtle movement towards dependency, where the professional 'takes over' with the tacit message, *trust me, I am a professional – do what I tell you and all will be well.'* And many people, feeling vulnerable and unsure of how best to proceed, fall gratefully into this trap, only to discover further down the line that they have been shortchanged by having their resilience, their expertise, their capacity to change and to take responsibility for their lives called into serious question. Maybe the professional worker did not intend this to happen; but by not practising the skills of partnership working this was the outcome.

It may be the case, of course, that in the early days of the professional relationship, the other person needs you to take some action on their behalf. A threat of immediate eviction, for example, is usually best removed, or at least delayed, by appropriate professional intervention. But if this is all that is done, and the person then walks away with a sigh of relief, they will soon discover that the 'evil day' returns once more to haunt them. As a worker you need to establish a trusting relationship where the real issues and problems are identified, and a clear strategy devised to help the person deal with them.

You can then begin to suggest to people that they are the experts in their own lives; that they know what is best for them and their family; that they know what needs to be done. If you can begin to articulate these issues, then your role as a professional will be to encourage, to support, to provide information, and to work with them to help them effect the changes which will be necessary if they are to emerge from their current cluster of problems. If you do all the work, and the person in difficulties remains a grateful but passive spectator, the chances are that whatever caused the problems will recur.

The skill in this approach is not just in the words and gestures that you use, but in your essential value-base, to ensure that respect and dignity are accorded to the other person in every possible way.

Exercise 2

Put yourself in the position of going to someone for help with a difficult problem. How would you like to be treated? What would partnership working mean for you? How would you feel if you were not treated in this way?

Passing the 'abducted by aliens' test

This somewhat tongue-in-cheek, light-hearted title refers to the importance of accurate accessible recording. Parker (2004: 116) uses this idea to capture an important issue, which he describes as follows:

If you were abducted by aliens tomorrow, would someone else in the office or agency be able to pick up your work and understand it?

The implications for assessment are clear. No matter how well you have worked in partnership with your service user, if this is not fully, accurately and clearly recorded there is a chance that all will be lost. Professional people-workers often lament the bureaucracy of paperwork and endless reports, but in truth they are the mechanisms for recording important work and for ensuring that others have access to it. Records and reports are often also essential before decisions can be taken by managers to allocate resources.

This means that you need to record all relevant information clearly, succinctly, in plain English, and state clearly where decisions need to be taken. Recommendations should also be clearly indicated. Most agencies, of course, have standard documents and proformas for recording information, and it is important that these are used properly. With multi-agency working becoming increasingly important, the need for accurate recording is paramount.

One further aspect of this is the right of access to information which service users, carers, patients and clients now have to their records. You need to be clear in your own mind what is your agency policy concerning access to records, and to make sure that you keep this in mind when completing your reports. It is best practice to share assessment documents with your service user, and for them to sign them and to have copies, although you will need first to check your agency policy.

Exercise 3

Try the 'abducted by alien' test either on some of your own records, or with another colleague, by exchanging records and giving each other feedback on them.

The Assessment Framework

One further aspect of assessment concerns working with children and families. In 2000 the Department of Health produced its *Framework for the Assessment of Children in Need and their Families*. This is required reading for anyone working with children and families in a professional context. The report states clearly that:

> Assessing whether a child is in need and the nature of these needs requires a systematic approach which uses the same framework or conceptual map for gathering and analysing information about all children and their families, but discriminates effectively between different types and levels of need ... It requires a thorough understanding of the developmental needs of children; the capacities of parents or caregivers to respond appropriately to those needs, and the impact of wider family and environmental factors on parenting capacity and children. (2000: 17)

In exploring these issues the report produced its assessment framework triangle, which indicates the range of issues that need to be taken into account in safeguarding and promoting the welfare of a child. The three arms of the triangle are (1) the child's developmental needs; (2) parenting capacity; and (3) family and environmental factors. It is only when all of these factors have been taken into account that a holistic assessment can be made. In this respect, the framework reflects the key skills and issues we have highlighted in this discussion, and underlines their importance for the assessment process.

Exercise 4

Obtain a copy of the Assessment Framework and study carefully the assessment triangle with its various components. Chapter two provides a detailed discussion of what is involved, and deserves careful study.

Final thoughts

Assessment is one of the most important tasks any professional worker can undertake. If it is done thoroughly by using the range of skills that is required, it can prove to be a most effective and empowering experience for everyone concerned. But it must be done properly and to the best of your ability.

References and Further reading

Coulshed, V. and Orme, J. (1998) *Social Work Practice: An Introduction*. 3nd edition. Basingstoke: Macmillan/BASW.

Department of Health (2000) *Framework for the Assessment of Children in Need and their Families*. DoH; DfEE; Home Office: The Stationery Office.

Hopkins, G. (1998) *Plain English for Social Services: A Guide to Better Communication*. Lyme Regis: Russell House Publishing.

Parker, J. (2004) *Effective Practice Learning in Social Work*. Exeter: Learning Matters.

Thompson, N. (2005) *Understanding Social Work*. 2nd edition. Basingstoke: Palgrave Macmillan.

Trevithick, P. (2005) *Social Work Skills – A Practice Handbook*. Maidenhead: Open University Press.

Related concepts   Empathy; establishing a professional relationship; partnership working.

Barrier Gestures

A barrier gesture is any action, behaviour or physical arrangement (such as room layout) that discourages the other person from feeling comfortable, thereby reducing their ability to communicate positively and effectively.

There are some situations, of course, where physical barriers are both sensible and necessary for the protection of the worker. There are classic examples of this within the prison service and how arrangements can be made for the safety of visitors. But many reception areas for public services have from time to time employed security screens in the hope of discouraging violence or abusive behaviour and for the protection of staff. These have not always worked, however, and have sometimes given the message that violent behaviour is being expected. Some people find such screens to be so impersonal that they provoke a suspicious, even aggressive, response. They much prefer to create an open, warm and human environment that respects the individual and encourages them in turn to behave respectfully towards the worker.

Exercise 1

Think of some situations and settings you know where there are security screens or similar barriers in operation. Do you think they are effective? Are they perhaps counter-productive by giving an expectation that some people may be violent? Are there better ways of counteracting violence?

People-workers also need to give careful thought to how furniture is arranged within the rooms and spaces where they meet with people and interview them. They need to give due attention to what seems open, welcoming and conducive to good shared communication, but not to overlook health and safety risk factors. These will include ensuring that:

- the worker can leave the room easily and quickly in case of difficulty
- panic buttons are visible and accessible but not 'in your face', and

- that decorative objects are not easily available to use as weapons or missiles.

Room layout communicates something to those who use the room, both in being welcome and open, but also in reinforcing boundaries for behaviour that is deemed unacceptable and that might put people at risk. Posters about behaviour, and the type of actions and language that are not acceptable, are also further examples of the ways in which boundaries can be clearly established.

The way in which professional workers, including doctors and solicitors, arrange their offices is also instructive. Do they sit powerfully behind a desk to enhance their status and power? Or do they sit sideways so that they are more accessible to people who come to see them?

All of the above are examples of a broad understanding of what barrier gestures involve, sometimes in emphasising or minimising the power differential between professionals and those who use their services, and sometimes in establishing the boundaries of what is acceptable conduct. The message is clear: go beyond this barrier and you are in trouble.

Non-verbal barrier gestures

More generally, however, within a wide range of people-work activities, barrier gestures are deemed to be unhelpful and discouraging to good communication. Sometimes these are very significant and obvious; other examples may seem more trivial and irritating. The overall impact of a barrier gesture upon the other person, however, is the message that we are not paying full attention to them, or even that we do not really want to hear what they have to say.

Some examples of barrier gestures which workers have been known to use, consciously or unconsciously, include:

- sitting with arms firmly crossed over the chest = a very defensive 'don't come near me' approach
- sitting slumped in the chair = I'm too 'chilled out' to be bothered with you
- fiddling with a book, pen or other object = this is a really interesting object I have got here and I prefer playing with this rather than listening to you
- jangling your keys and change in your pocket = I'll be glad to get away from here into my car or to do some serious shopping
- fiddling with your hair, or ears, or face = I'm feeling rather uneasy with this conversation and need to engage in some self-comforting activity

- gazing out of the window = there are far more interesting things happening out there than in this interview
- glancing at your watch surreptitiously = I'll be glad when this interview is over
- answering phone calls during the interview = this person is not important enough for me to give them uninterrupted time – see how busy and important I am though
- Placing yourself behind the desk = now, little person, what can I do for you today – see how important I am and how lucky you are to have me to talk to.

The interpretations given to each of these barrier gestures are perhaps tongue-in-cheek and slightly exaggerated, but they make a serious point. There are a number of things we can do during an interview that can be off-putting to the other person, and give a message that we are not 100 per cent interested in what they have to say to us. Some barrier gestures we can perhaps easily identify and rectify, but we all have our idiosyncracies that we are hardly aware of. Little mannerisms, which in themselves really do not matter much and may in some situations be rather endearing, but which in a professional interview could be irritating and off-putting. The only way of spotting these, of course, is either to ask permission for a trusted colleague to sit in with you and give you feedback, or in a training context to video yourself in an interview, and watch yourself afterwards in action.

The reason for stressing this is not to make you too self-conscious so that you become wooden, unnatural and awkward – exactly the opposite. It is to help you focus totally, warmly and openly on the other person, and to remove anything which distracts from enabling them to feel they have been fully listened to and accepted.

Reading the signs

This awareness, of course, will help you to deal with barrier gestures that service users or clients use when being interviewed by you. In the discussion on non-verbal communication it is argued that all of us communicate non-verbally all the time through our body language. Just as we need as people-workers to be aware of what we are communicating to our service users through our body language, so too we can learn to 'read the signs' from other people's body language, so that we can appreciate what they are trying to say to us without necessarily being able to put it into words.

Exercise 2

Revisit the list of barrier gestures and responses outlined above and try 'turning the tables'. If the service user or client uses these gestures, what messages do you think they are trying to convey to us?

The skills for people-workers lie in our ability to read the signs accurately, and to respond in ways that help to draw the other person into the interview, and not drive a deeper wedge between you. It is helpful, therefore, to be able to put into words what you suspect the barrier gestures are communicating to you. For example:

J, I can see from how you are sitting that you don't really want to be here.

I guess, J, that if I were in your shoes I would want to be somewhere else right now.

Tell me if I have got it wrong, J, but you seem pretty angry and fed up to me.

Feeling bored, J?

J, how can I help you get a bit more out of our time together today?

Sometimes, however, we can misunderstand other people's gestures. For example, in some cultures it is a sign of respect to someone in authority not to maintain eye contact with them. If this were to be misinterpreted as being disrespectful, a serious breakdown in communication could well follow.

Mirroring

One of the skills which sometimes works to help unlock someone's barrier gestures is called mirroring. Stated simply, this approach suggests that as the worker you mirror the gestures which the other person is using – for example, if they are sitting with arms firmly crossed, you do the same for a while. And then, as you talk to them, slowly begin to unfold your arms, and you may find that they copy your actions and begin visibly to relax. It is worth an occasional try, but it needs to be done subtly, and there is no guarantee that it will work.

Tricky moments

There will be occasions when there can be no doubt what the person is feeling. You may be faced with someone who raises a hand or shakes a fist at you, or who suddenly stands over you in a threatening manner. Your personal safety may well then be at risk, and you will need to decide how best to respond. It is easy to say 'stay calm' when your insides have turned to jelly and you feel weak at the knees, but if you can display an outward appearance of calmness and of not being intimidated, this will help. Initially, you should try to defuse the situation by saying something like:

> J, I know you are angry and upset, but please stop doing that.
>
> J, please sit down – it does not help either of us if you try to threaten me.
>
> J, I can't help you if you treat me like this.
>
> J, violence doesn't solve anything J – it really doesn't – please sit down.

If the situation escalates, then the time for talking is over, and you need to leave the room as quickly as possible and summon help. Your safety is paramount.

Final thoughts

There are, of course, no guarantees that you will break through the barriers which are being erected, but at least if you can begin to put into words what you suspect they are feeling it will go some way towards helping them realise that they are being listened to and respected.

Further reading

Thompson, N. (2003) *Communication and Language – A Handbook of Theory and Practice*. Basingstoke: Palgrave Macmillan.
Trevithick, P. (2005) *Social Work Skills – A Practice Handbook*. 2nd edition. Maidenhead: Open University Press.

Related concepts   Empathy; non-verbal communication.

Breaking Bad News

If there is one thing arguably more difficult than receiving bad news, it is having to break bad news to someone. If you have ever had to do this, you will know how distressing it can be for the 'breaker' and the receiver. Your stomach churns as the moment approaches; you worry about how the person will react; you wonder how it would be if the situation were in reverse; and perhaps memories of bad news you have received in the past come flooding back. Without doubt, this is not territory you would choose to be in.

But sometimes, as part of our job as people-workers, we are called upon to undertake this important but painful task. And while there are no easy golden rules to guarantee that such occasions will go well, there are some guidelines to help you that are set out below.

It is helpful first of all, however, to explore some of the situations where as a professional you may be called on to break bad news. There are occasions when you may have to tell someone that:

- you are taking their child into care
- their relative has died
- they have a terminal illness
- they are being made redundant
- their teenage son has been arrested
- they cannot receive the services they had hope for.

Exercise 1

The list outlined above provided just a few examples. Spend a few moments adding to it both from your own experience in your work setting, and from likely scenarios that you know other colleagues have had to deal with.

Exercise 2

Look again at your list. Try to identify what it is that worries you most about having to break bad news. Jot your thoughts down before you move onto the next section of this discussion.

You have now set the scene for exploring this difficult aspect of communication skills. The section that follows outlines a way of approaching such situations in an appropriate professional manner, which puts the other person's needs 'in the driving seat', but also helps you best prepare. You do not need telling that the news you are about to break will come as a shock; you cannot disguise that, nor minimise the impact it will have upon that person. What you can do, however, is to remember that, if you do your best and follow the guidelines we suggest, you will earn the gratitude of that person (in due course, if not straightaway) for the way you have handled it. How you deal with this situation *will* make a difference to the person receiving the news.

Breaking bad news – preparation

Although you may or may not know the person to whom you are going to break bad news well enough to predict how they will respond – they may get very distressed; or go into themselves in a protective silence, for example – you know yourself well enough to know that good preparation is important for you if you are going to stand even a chance of doing it well. Preparation is important at the 'head level' and at the 'heart level'.

Head-level preparation

'Head-level' preparation is about being as sure as you can be concerning the information you are going to be asked about, when you have broken the bad news. Try to put yourself into their shoes and anticipate what their questions might be; find out in advance as much information as you can. This will involve being very clear about what you do know and can find out about, and what questions will have to remain unanswered. For example, if you are breaking news about a person involved in an accident or in a serious medical condition, there may well be many things which you do not know about, and which may be beyond your professional expertise anyway. In such situations, you must be honest and say you do not know; but you may be able to suggest other colleagues who will be able to provide these important answers.

There is another set of difficult questions, however, that no one will ever be able to answer fully, and these are the big 'Why?' questions that people often ask in moments of profound shock. Frequently, these questions pose deep existential concerns for that person's worldview, which may be on the brink of disintegration in the face of such bad news. For example:

- Why did God allow this to happen?
- Why did God take this person away and leave me?

- What have I done to deserve this?
- Why should it have happened to him/her – he/she was such a lovely person?

These and many other searching questions brook no easy answer, but, nevertheless, can place the breaker of bad news in a difficult situation. It is worth some prior thought, therefore, to prepare yourself for responding to such painful, challenging moments. This is important whether or not you yourself belong to a faith community or believe in God, Allah or a Supreme Being. It is tempting sometimes, for example, to offer someone in distress an insight into your own world-view in the hope that it will comfort them in their moment of anguish. A devout Christian or Muslim, for instance, may believe that whatever happens must somehow be the will and purpose of God or Allah. 'Insch Allah' is how Muslims would express this: it is God's will. By definition, there can be nothing that happens that cannot fall outside the will and purpose of the Divine Being. But to state this to a person who has no such belief could be to alienate them from you at the very moment when you have the opportunity as another human being to be open and supportive to them. By contrast, the person who has received the bad news may have a faith which can accommodate this disaster, and tells you so, but you may feel appalled by this world-view to which you would feel totally unable to subscribe yourself. Then there are the searching questions for people who belong to a faith community but whose belief in God is shattered by the awful news they have just received. They may ask you how they will be able to cope from now on.

The variations are endless, but in many ways the issue for you is the same. Whatever your own world-view is; whether or not you subscribe to a religious faith; no matter how painful or upsetting you may find the scenario to be personally, your principal responsibility is to the person who has just received the news you have brought to them. It is not for you to bring your own 'agenda' into play with how you do, or do not, view the world, and whether you do or do not have a religious faith. Your task is to be as open as possible to the hurt, the anguish and the confusion that the person is experiencing. Easy answers are a misnomer: they are not answers, and they are usually offered to make *you* feel better, not the person you are working with.

The most helpful responses, therefore, will be the ones that treat the other person with the utmost seriousness and respect; that listen to their pain and distress and do not seek to offer trite statements, however well-intentioned; and which seek to 'hear the music beyond the words' when such questions are posed. In other words, if you can respond to, and acknowledge the pain and confusion that these questions represent, you may be far more helpful because the person begins to feel that you really are listening to them, and have begun to realise the depth of their loss.

Heart-level preparation

These issues have already brought us into the second aspect of preparation, the 'heart-level' or emotional preparation. It is important that any disquiet, nervousness or even fear at having to undertake such a task as breaking bad news does not get in the way. Nor must you allow your own distress or upset to intrude into the interview or meeting which you are about to conduct. In other words, you need to take your emotional temperature, and talk through with someone you can trust how you are feeling about this task. Far better to do your crying as part of your own preparation than let your own emotions spill over into the interview when you are having to deal with the tears of the other person. But even if it is not likely to reduce you to tears, it is still important to talk through with someone else how you are going to handle the situation; what words you are going to use to break the bad news, and how you will seek to respond to some of the issues which inevitably will arise.

This is not to say that everything will go as you have planned – far from it – but you will be surprised how much better you will handle the encounter if you have taken the trouble to do some of this important preparation in advance.

One further tip: it is useful to jot down some key information to leave with the person you are going to see. The chances are that they will be in shock and will not remember details very well. If you have left information for them in writing, including some contact details for yourself or others, that will be a great help. But you will need to give careful thought to what you write down.

Breaking bad news – planning for the meeting

Much of what follows is based on a protocol for breaking bad news developed to help medical professionals in their roles, but it is relevant and easily adaptable to other people-work contexts. The SPIKES protocol was originally developed by Baile and Buckman (2000), and you will find it helpful to consider the issues they raise when you are involved in breaking bad news yourself.

S: the setting

It clearly makes a big difference to the interview or meeting as to where it takes place. If it is to be in your own office, you will have far more control over what happens. You will be able to ensure a private uninterrupted space, where the phone is on 'divert' and staff know you are not to be interrupted. You will be able to ensure that a box of tissues and refreshments are available, and that the layout of the room is appropriate.

You may find, however, that you are having to conduct this discussion in a less favourable setting. You may have to break bad news to someone in a hospital ward, or in a day or residential setting; or visiting someone in prison where you have far less control over the environment you will be working in. It is important, therefore, to do everything in your power to seek a private room to conduct this interview. Contact the staff in advance; explain that you have some sensitive issues to explore, and that you will need privacy. This will be especially important if the person has hearing difficulties: you will not want to have to raise your voice to impart such difficult news. But if privacy cannot be guaranteed, you will need to think about how to position yourself so that you can speak in as quiet a voice as possible during the interview.

If you are breaking bad news in someone's home, there are other considerations to bear in mind. One distinct advantage is that the person will be on home territory, and will not have to make the journey back from your office to their home after hearing the news. But home territory brings other hazards. Music, pets, television, other people being present, children, casual callers, phone calls: all of these can impact upon the meeting you are trying to conduct. Again, you will need to introduce the reason for your visit early on, and if need be invite the person to prepare themselves appropriately. You may need to ask for the TV be turned off. It is not your territory, but do try to take some control so that you have a reasonable chance of doing your difficult job effectively.

Sometimes the setting will be a telephone call, and this too needs careful thought. You will be surprised perhaps by the sheer volume of information that your tone of voice can convey over the phone. If you do not believe that, then think about occasions when you have been expecting news (good or bad) to be conveyed to you by telephone. The chances are that you will sense the outcome of the phone call in the first few seconds, simply by the tone of voice of the person making the call, and how they go about the task of talking to you. If you are using the phone to make an urgent appointment to visit someone to break bad news face to face, you will need to decide how much to say to them in advance. If you make it sound too light and 'come day, go day', they will not be at all prepared for what you have to say; if you do manage to convey the seriousness of the situation, you may find yourself giving most, if not all of the information in that phone call, especially as they will inevitably ask you questions about why you want to pay them a visit. Here again, preparation about what you will say and how you will say it are invaluable. If you do have to tell them the news over the phone, you will need to ask them if they have anyone with them: are they sitting down, because you have some bad news for them.

Finally, you may find that, as often is the case with the police, you are having to 'cold call'. Unlike the police, however, where the unexpected visit from uniformed officers immediately conveys some important information, this may be not be the case with you. Again, you need to be prepared, with a form of words to use which deals sensitively but clearly with the reason for your visit. Also, you must ensure that you have your ID card or badge with you so that they know they are receiving a visit from a bona fide worker.

P: the other person's perspective

You will have had time to rehearse what you need to say and how you are going to handle the meeting. But for the person on the receiving end, this could be a bolt out of the blue for which they are completely unprepared. In such situations it is likely that they will not take in the news you are giving to them. It is important, therefore, that you try to assess the person's perceptions, and how they seem to be absorbing and understanding what you are seeking to convey. Their reaction may suggest that they have not fully appreciated the seriousness of what you are telling them. It is helpful, therefore, to go over the ground as many times as is necessary, if need be by asking them to 'play back' to you the key features. As mentioned in the section on preparation, it is useful to have some key information available to give to them in writing, as they may be in shock for a while and unable to take in fully what you are saying.

I: invitation

Another issue to bear in mind is that all professionals have their own jargon which they use as easily and at times as unthinkingly as drawing breath. With the best will in the world and with every intention to communicate clearly, you may still sometimes fail to guard against this when talking to people. This means that you must be prepared to go over the ground more than once, and to invite them to ask questions if they feel they have not fully understood some of the terms you have used. 'There is no such thing as a silly question' is a very useful golden rule to share with them.

Sometimes, of course, further information is not always appropriate. The person may feel they have got enough to deal with and do not want to know any more, at least as far as the immediate moment is concerned. In medical contexts, there is often the issue of the extent to which people understand the full implications of a medical diagnosis, but other professionals have similar situations to deal with, where people may not always fully appreciate the implications of what is being told them. It is important, therefore, to leave the invitation open; to invite people to think about what has been said, and to jot down any issues that they may wish to ask you about next time you meet.

K: knowledge

How you convey information to the person is important; the timing of it, and how you control the flow of information can make all the difference between a successful and unsuccessful interview. As an example of this, think about meeting with an insurance sales representative, or a double-glazing salesperson. How often have such interviews led to the potential buyer feeling bamboozled, and totally confused by information overload? They reach a point where they find it impossible even to ask a sensible question, and just long for the meeting to end so that they can catch their breath. This is the worst possible scenario for you to emulate when breaking bad news.

It is important, therefore, to convey information in bite-sized chunks which the person can understand, and which you can easily check out as the interview unfolds. This is a major communication skill because it requires you to be aware of how the person is absorbing information. You want to avoid going too slowly, which can feel patronising, or too swiftly, which can feel insensitive. Finding the 'middle way' is the key to a successful interview, and this will be different for each person you work with. The main point always to bear in mind, therefore, is that the imparting of information is only half the story: how it is received and understood is the other half, and if you do not take responsibility for checking this other half of the equation, you will not have done your job at all well.

E: explore emotions and empathise

How someone receives the information you are giving to them will often be indicated by, and measured by, their emotional response. It is important, therefore, that you have prepared yourself to deal with this aspect of the interview in a sensitive way. Sometimes the immediate bursting into tears is easier to deal with than someone going into an impenetrable silence. But even tears can be challenging, especially if there are gender issues involved. Not all men find it easy to cry; some more readily express an angry response. Some people find it difficult to be with men who are able to cry; occasionally it stimulates upset or distress within us. The skill of saying nothing while the person expresses their tearfulness or anger should not be underestimated. It is helpful sometimes simply to acknowledge to them that you realise how painful this is for them, and that you are not trying to rush them through such an emotional response to the news you have broken. Just to say to them that you realise that this news will inevitably have been deeply upsetting and disturbing, will be a small step towards achieving a degree of empathy with them. And to have someone perceptive and sensitive enough to stay with them during these emotional moments can make all the difference to how they deal with things subsequently.

S: strategy and summary

Interviews need to come to an end, and how this type of interview concludes is very much up to your skill and judgment, and how much time you have allowed for the meeting. There is always the chance, of course, that in a person's home the end of the interview may be precipitated by a child bursting into the room, or the dog creating a diversion, or the phone ringing. But even so you will want to ensure that the meeting closes in as caring and planned a way as possible. You do not want to be walking away when the person is still deeply distressed.

You need to have a strategy, therefore, for dealing with what needs to happen next. This may involve contacting other professionals; arranging a further meeting; fixing a time when you will ring them to see how they are. In extreme cases you may need to contact medical services to arrange for an assessment or other medical intervention. It is always useful to offer a brief, sensitive summary of the story so far, and what you have agreed to do next, and to leave information in writing, especially any important contact details.

Exercise 3

Revisit some of the scenarios you identified in Exercises 1 and 2. Make some notes about what sort of preparation you would need to undertake in order to be as ready as possible to deal with the issues. Then use the SPIKES protocol to produce further notes on how you would intend to achieve best practice when dealing with the person concerned.

Final thoughts

As we indicated at the outset, there are so many different scenarios for breaking bad news that it is impossible to think about, let alone plan for, every eventuality. What can be said, however, is that in breaking bad news it will be your approach, your values and your personality as a worker that will shine through clearest of all. If you develop the skills to do it well, you will earn the gratitude of those you work with more than you will perhaps ever realise.

There can be no denying that such work is stressful and at times upsetting. It is no disgrace to feel emotionally drained after such an encounter, or to find that you have suddenly become 'weepy' afterwards. It is crucial, therefore, to take good care of yourself, personally and professionally, by finding an appropriate person to talk to afterwards, to offload and to get back into shape emotionally to work with other people.

References and Further reading

Baile, W.F. and Buckman, R. (2000) 'SPIKES: a six step protocol for delivering bad news', *The Oncologist*, vol. 5 (4): 302–311. (online via www.theoncologist.alphamedpress.org)

Buckman, R. (1996) *I Don't Know What to Say*. London: Pan Books.

Related concepts   Active listening; empathy; non-verbal communication; religion; spirituality; supervision.

Chairing Meetings

An increasingly important communication skill for anyone involved with people-work is that of chairing meetings. Meetings themselves are channels of communication, both for those physically present and participating in the discussion and decision making, and also for those not attending who may need to discover what was decided by accessing the minutes.

Whether the meetings are fairly low-key, or of huge significance such as a case conference, some of the principles and issues are the same when it comes to the task of chairing them successfully.

Exercise 1

Spend some time in a meeting you are involved with as a participant trying to identify how well the chair of the meeting does the job. What seems to make it go well? What does the chair do, or not do? How involved do the participants seem to be? Are there any frustrating aspects of the meeting? If so, what are they? How would you handle it differently?

Guidelines and principles

In fact, chairing a meeting is not all that difficult if you keep certain guidelines and principles firmly in mind. One of the most important of these is preparation.

Preparation

There are some basic points to remember before any meeting takes place. These include:

- Why is the meeting necessary? What purpose(s) will it fulfil?
- Who needs to be present in order for the meeting to be effective and purposeful?

- What are the desired outcomes from the meeting?
- What is a good time to hold the meeting? How much advance notice will people require in order to be able to attend?
- Where is the best place to hold it ?
- What considerations must be made to enable participants to participate fully? For example, will you need a loop system, or a palantypist or interpreter to be present? Does the date clash with religious festivals or prayer times?
- What information needs to be circulated to participants before the meeting in order for them to come prepared?
- Who will take the notes/minutes of the meeting and see to their distribution?
- What amount of time is available for the meeting? When should it end?

Preparing the agenda

It is important for you, as chair, to be very familiar with the shape and structure of the meeting, the order of the items, and what actions or decisions are needed to flow from them.

If there are some difficult or contentious issues to be discussed, organise the agenda in such a way as to allow enough time. You may wish to allocate blocks of time for certain items. For example, you could suggest that after the first 30 minutes you will move to the substantive item for discussion. This is a matter of judgment and prior thought on your part as the chair, with prior consultation with other members as appropriate.

It is also worth annotating your own copy of the agenda with various points that you need to remember as the meeting progresses.

The meeting itself

Many of the skills you will need successfully to chair a meeting are the same ones you need in your one-to-one interactions and interviews; it is just that they need to be adapted to a larger group setting. For example, you will want at the outset to ensure that you begin punctually, and indicate how long the meeting is likely to last. You will need to introduce yourself and give any additional information about yourself that confirms your appropriateness as the chair of the meeting. You will then need to remind people of the purpose of the meeting, and what they are hoping to achieve.

Next, you need to invite people to introduce themselves and the capacity in which they are attending the meeting. This serves two functions: first, it enables everyone present to put faces to names; and second, it highlights the roles and responsibilities the agencies represented have to fulfil. In days of increasing multi-agency cooperation, this is particularly important.

Matters arising are important. There may be action points from the previous meeting that need to be reported upon, and the outcome noted in the minutes. It is your responsibility as chair to identify these, and to ask the appropriate person to give a brief report on progress.

When you reach the substantive items on the agenda for discussion, you need to have a clear view about what outcome you are seeking to achieve. This will affect how you chair the meeting. For example, if the item is a free-flowing exchange of ideas about various ways in which the organisation can improve its image and profile with the general public, you may want people to have brief discussions in pairs to get them going, and report their ideas back to the whole group. You may then want to suggest that a sub-group brings a considered set of recommendations to the next meeting.

By contrast, if there is a serious matter to be decided at the meeting itself, you will need to consider how best it should be introduced. It may be right for you to speak briefly about it, highlighting the arguments for and against; or you may have invited someone else in advance to do this for you. Whatever tactic you adopt, it is important that you ensure that all points of view are clearly articulated in the discussion. Inevitably, some members may be more vociferous than others, so you will need from time to time to invite those who have not yet spoken to share their views with the meeting. You may do this in a general way, or speak directly to someone and ask them if they have anything they wish to add to the discussion. This needs to be done in a sensitive way, but you need to be seen as a chair who is even-handed and values the contribution which everyone can make to the debate.

Undoubtedly, one of the most difficult skills to learn is how to keep a discussion focused. It is your task as chair to keep the discussion on track without appearing rude or domineering yourself. If you do not do this, there is bound to be a growing feeling that the real purpose of the meeting is not being achieved. One useful trick of the trade is to thank people for their contributions so far, and to remind them of what the main issues are that they need to decide, and to draw their attention to aspects of the topic that have not yet been discussed. Towards the end, you can ask if anyone else wishes to contribute before you call for a vote. In extreme cases you will need to be very assertive and to remind people of the ground rules whereby they agree to listen to each other without interruption, and no one attempts to be domineering. On occasion, you may need to address the person who is being domineering, and thank them for making their point so clearly, but asking them to sit back for a while to allow other members to put their points forward.

You may also be surprised about how effective some appropriate hand gestures can be. If you look clearly at someone whom you wish to invite to speak and point to them, and simply hold your other hand up in the direction of the person whom you want to stay quiet, you are giving a message about your authority as chair.

Your role as chair also involves keeping an eye on the clock. When you feel that the issues have been sufficiently aired, announce that you intend to take the vote very soon. This helps people focus their thoughts on the key themes of the debate, and also provides a final opportunity for anyone who has not yet contributed to have their say.

Voting

You need to record carefully those who vote FOR; those who vote AGAINST; and those who ABSTAIN. You should then formally announce the decision of the meeting. You must be aware, however, of any constitutional regulations in this matter. Some organisations constitutionally require a 75 per cent majority in favour, for example, before any major change can be implemented. The meeting should be reminded of such regulations at the outset of the discussion and before the vote is taken. If it is a large meeting, you may wish to appoint two tellers to take responsibility for counting the votes.

Another point to bear in mind is who is eligible to vote. There are some organisations where there is a strict membership with the entitlement to vote, and there needs to be a mechanism to ensure that non-voting people at the meeting clearly understand this rule. This is sometimes achieved by issuing voting papers, especially in cases where people are being elected to office.

The nightmare scenario for any chair, of course, is an evenly balanced vote. Sometimes the chair is allowed an additional casting vote, and it may be important that you exercise this. However, there is wisdom in thinking twice before you do this. Sometimes it is better simply to note that the meeting is so divided that you will need to return to the discussion next time. But there will be times when you will have to cast that deciding vote. If you do take that course of action, you should state your reasons for your decision. It is not easy or comfortable territory, but the chair has to fulfil this role effectively if business is to be conducted in due order.

Involving service users and carers in meetings

One further area demands particular skills from you as chair. Increasingly, there are meetings within health and social care settings when service users and carers are involved in discussions and debates with professionals about their welfare, and the resources that are allocated to them. In such situations, as chair you will need to ensure, in advance of the meeting, that mentors or advocates will attend to support service users and carers who might feel intimidated by a powerful array of professionals.

Your role as chair is crucial in welcoming people and helping to put them at ease. You will need to remind them that specific time and space will be given to listening to their point of view, both directly and if necessary through their advocate. You will want everyone to feel that this is a genuine commitment, so that, whatever the outcome, they will feel that they have been properly listened to and their concerns fully heard.

Of course, there will be occasions when the service users have no hesitation in voicing their concerns angrily and vociferously at the meeting. Your role then will be to encourage them directly, and with the support of their advocate if need be, to listen to what others also have to say. This is not easy; sometimes you may need to adjourn the meeting for a five or ten minute 'comfort break' to allow tempers to calm down, and for you to speak to people informally. If, however, you can identify the fears and concerns that underlie people's contributions to the discussion, it will go a long way to helping the meeting come to its decision. If everyone respects your calm and authoritative role as chair, it will help them move to a successful conclusion.

Endings

It is important when you enter 'injury time' in a meeting – this is the period of about 15 minutes before its scheduled time for completion – that you draw people's attention to the time, and to the items still remaining for discussion. It is helpful sometimes to check to see if people can stay a further 30 minutes to complete the agenda. If they can, well and good, and you need to respect that revised timetable. If, however, people have to leave, then you need to agree what can be left until next time.

Any other business?

There are various approaches to the mysterious item on many agendas: *Any Other Business* (AOB). As chair you will need to exercise some judgment about any items that are raised. If they are fairly straightforward and can be dealt with in the time remaining, then there is no reason why you should not deal with them there and then. But if they require longer debate, or appear to be contentious or even mischievous, you should rule that they be placed on the agenda for the next meeting so that people have adequate notice.

59

Date of the next meeting

It is not unusual for the trickiest discussion to focus around the date for the next meeting. If you are involved in a committee which has to meet regularly throughout the year, it is helpful to set the dates for the next six or so meetings well in advance.

Before you close the meeting formally, remember to thank people for their attendance and their contributions.

Debriefing

If chairing meetings is still new to you, you may well find it helpful to have a debriefing discussion with a more experienced colleague to identify what went well, and to feed back ways in which you might have handled certain parts of the meeting differently. This will help you develop your confidence.

You will also find that you are beginning to watch other people's skills and techniques in chairing meetings where you are a participant. It is good to have some role models to help you develop your own particular skills, and it can be reassuring to see how even experienced chairs can, from time to time, struggle in this role.

Finally, you need to arrange to meet with the person taking the minutes to ensure that they are accurate and ready in time to send out to members before the next meeting.

Minute taking

Many organisations have secretarial support for this task, but from time to time you may be called upon to fulfil this role. It goes without saying that the accuracy of minutes and notes of meetings is of vital importance. People who lead busy lives and attend many meetings may well not remember the details of the discussions and the decisions taken at each one, so the record of the meeting is crucial. For committees and groups which meet on a regular basis, these ongoing records are the only means whereby the story of what is decided is accurately told. Future members of the committee may need to look back on the minutes from several years back to check certain facts and decisions. So the minutes need to be accurate, agreed by the committee meeting members, and stored safely but accessibly, in hard copy as well as electronically, for all who have good reason to consult them.

Final thoughts

This discussion has highlighted the importance of good communication skills in the context of chairing meetings and recording the decisions and outcomes. If as chair you can develop the necessary communication skills to help people work together in meetings to debate difficult issues and come to clear decisions, you will have made a significant contribution to the organisations involved.

Further reading

Hawkins, C. (1997) *First Aid for Meetings*. Oregon: Bookpartners Inc.

Honey, P. (2004) *How to Chair Meetings Effectively*. Maidenhead: Peter Honey Publications Ltd.

Kelsey, D., Plumb, P. and Kippy, R. (2003) *Great Meetings: How to Facilitate Like a Pro*. Maine: Hanson Park Press.

Web based resource: Imperial College Union.ICU skills guide 2005–6. How to chair a meeting effectively www.union.ic.ac.uk (accessed Jan 2007)

Related concepts   Interpreters; feedback; non-verbal communication.

Challenging

The ability to challenge inappropriate or offensive language or behaviour in others is one of the most difficult of communication skills to put into practice. Often we feel caught between the 'rock' of doing or saying nothing and thereby appearing to collude with the other person; and the 'hard place' of over-reacting and making matters worse by provoking or alienating the other person and losing the thread of the discussion which you were trying to hold with them.

Part of the reason for this, perhaps, lies in the word itself. 'Challenging' seems to be a very aggressive activity, highly 'macho' and confrontational: very much 'in your face' as we might say. Certainly in some of the early examples of anti-racist awareness training an openly confrontational approach was often deemed necessary by some of the trainers in order to bring white people up with a jolt, and to realise just how serious and ingrained racism is within a white-dominated society. Many people-workers may feel very uncomfortable, however, about being expected to adopt such a style or approach, however worthy the intention might be; it seems to smack too much of adopting the moral high ground in our relationship with others.

Just because it is difficult, however, does not mean that you should give up the attempt. Challenging is an important activity for you because it goes to the very heart of the value-base of the work you undertake with others. The values of dignity, respect, social justice and celebrating diversity are central to your work, but they do not come automatically or easily, Indeed, they often need to be fought for against considerable opposition, as many events in the early part of the twenty-first century so eloquently testify. Challenging opposing sets of values is important precisely because of this struggle: if prejudice and discriminatory practice are not challenged, it is one further tiny victory for intolerance and bigotry.

> **Exercise 1**
>
> Spend a few moments jotting down some examples of statements or behaviour which you feel would be important for you to challenge. Keep these to hand while this discussion unfolds.

It is likely that your examples will feature some of the major social attitudes which have become contemporary 'isms': racism, sexism, classism, disablism, and heterosexism as well as homophobia. Characteristics and differences that are seen by some to enrich our society are regarded by others with fear, suspicion and hostility. That each and every individual is capable of acting badly towards others is a sad feature of our human existence: it is when groups of people are labelled as deviant or unacceptable simply by their belonging to that group, that we enter dangerous territory where the importance of challenging becomes imperative.

Styles of challenging

We need to state at the outset that for all its potentially aggressive potential, challenging as an activity can have quite a different 'feel' to it. It can be subtle, or gentle; it can draw on humour, or be accomplished non-verbally. Challenging, in other words, can often be achieved elegantly without the confrontation that many people so dislike.

Not all challenging is on a 'one-to-one' basis. Citizens Advice Bureaux, for example, have an important social policy arm whereby issues which arise from individual enquirers that are seen to affect larger numbers of people, are brought together into a campaigning activity. Pressure is brought to bear on local, or national government to raise their awareness, and to seek some amelioration. Other examples of pressure groups such as the Child Poverty Action Group and various homeless charities provide similar examples of ways in which challenging can be achieved through campaigning to improve the quality of people's lives.

On an individual level, several options are open to you when faced with language and behaviour which is offensive. The most straightforward approach is calmly but firmly to ask the person to stop behaving or speaking in this way because you find it unacceptable. You need to find the best form of words to use, of course, but if you can own the discomfort and upset which this causes it will enable you to challenge it. It is even more helpful if your organisation has a policy about such matters, when you can point this out to people and say that people are asked not to talk or behave like that when on your premises.

Challenging, however, is rarely straightforward. Sometimes, in the middle of a difficult interview, someone may use language that we find offensive. You may well feel, however, that to interrupt the flow of the interview by making an immediate challenge would be too disruptive to the main purpose of the interview. In such circumstances you may well simply make a mental note of this, and when the interview is winding down, gently refer to the incident, and ask the person not to talk like that with you again.

It is useful to have some responses already prepared, or at least thought through, so that you do not always have to struggle to find the best form of words to use. Some examples of this include:

- I don't think we can say that these days, do you?
- That really makes me feel uncomfortable when you say/do that.
- I can't agree with what you have just said.
- I don't think it is right to label everybody like that.
- When people come to this office we do ask everyone, including the staff, to be careful about the language we all use so that we don't cause offence.

The key issue is that you are not necessarily inviting a debate about the subject, although from time to time that may be helpful and appropriate, and will help you to discuss the value-base you are working from. The important thing is that you are making clear how you feel about their discriminatory or offensive language and behaviour; you are owning and acknowledging the negative impact it has on you; you are naming it, and are reinforcing the boundaries within which you find it acceptable to work with this person.

Many agencies have statements about language and behaviour clearly on view for everyone to see. For people who cannot read, other ways of putting this message across need to be found – pictorial representations are useful alternatives here. In the last resort you would be entitled to draw your meeting to a close and to refuse to work any further with the person if their offensive behaviour or language persisted. In such situations it is a good idea to warn them that you feel unable to continue, but to ask them to wait so that you can bring in your manager to reinforce the point and to support you. All being well, the person will then modify their behaviour, but if they do need to be excluded from the agency, then you will have had appropriate support for this course of action.

If you do need to take this drastic action, it is helpful to follow it up with a letter explaining the reason for your decision, and offering them a further appointment on the strict understanding that next time they will observe the ground-rules you have established. This gives them a chance to reflect and to make a fresh start next time.

Sometimes, of course, this sort of behaviour is the result of someone being heavily under the influence of alcohol or through drugs misuse. It is wise to call an early halt to any such interview, and ask them to return for a further appointment when they are in full control of themselves. You should not be expected to put yourself in a risky, vulnerable situation by continuing an interview with someone whose self-control is in question. Nor is it fair to expect a person who is not in full control of themselves to engage in discussion or work on key issues that affect their lives.

Exercise 2

Draw up a number of scenarios where you feel you would need to challenge someone, and make a list of possible responses. Then invite a colleague or your practice teacher to role play these so that you can practise these skills in a safe environment.

Final thoughts

'All it takes for evil to flourish is for good people to do nothing.' If we apply this principle to our present discussion we will see that even the smallest, very low-key challenge may make an important impact.

Further reading

Thompson, N. (2003) *Communication and Language: A Handbook of Theory and Practice*. Basingstoke: Palgrave Macmillan.
Trevithick, P. (2005) *Social Work Skills – A Practice Handbook*. Maidenhead: Open University Press. (pp. 237 ff)

Related concepts   Anti-discriminatory practice; barrier gestures; empathy; endings.

Clarifying

(*see* active listening)

Confidentiality

In almost all aspects of professional people-work the principle of confidentiality is highlighted as part of the value-base and the various codes of practice. If people feel that their privacy will be violated by the person they speak to, or their personal details made public in some way, they will not have confidence in the service they are being offered. Nor will the relationship that is being offered to them be regarded as professional. So it is extremely important that people are reassured at the outset about this central tenet of professional people-work: they need to know where they are before they can begin to trust the person they are working with.

This general principle, however, is not as straightforward as some would think.

Exercise 1

Think about the agency you work for, or an agency you are familiar with. What is said to your service users about confidentiality? What are the particular aspects of confidentiality which are central to your work? Are there any boundaries to confidentiality? If so, what are they, and how are these boundaries explained to people?

This exercise will have revealed that confidentiality is rarely, if ever, absolute. Agencies recognise that there are sometimes over-riding societal responsibilities laid upon them which would mean that an individual's right to confidentiality must be compromised. For example, if information is divulged which indicates that a vulnerable person – a child or an adult – is being put at risk, or is being abused or harmed in any way, then there is a duty laid upon the worker to report that information. This would be done first of all within the agency to an appropriate senior manager, and then if necessary to another agency such as the police or social services who are charged with a role of protecting vulnerable people.

This has been a topic which has posed a particular challenge for leaders in faith-based organisations, where traditionally the 'priest's confessional'(or its equivalent) has been absolute. In recent years, however, there has been an increasing awareness of the over-riding duty to protect vulnerable children in particular, and faith groups have been keen to ensure that their policies and practices respect this moral imperative.

One fundamental point to stress is that confidentiality is both an organisational as well as an individual commitment. From the individual worker's perspective there is a commitment that information will not be divulged to other people outside the organisation except in very exceptional circumstances. But this commitment does not mean that the information will not be shared within the organisation: it is of crucial importance that the managers are aware of what is happening, so that they can advise the worker on the best action to take, especially if sensitive information is being handled.

This book focuses on communication skills, and does not attempt a full-scale discussion of complex issues which can be found elsewhere in the literature. The key challenge for people-workers with this topic, therefore, is how most effectively the topic of confidentiality can be raised with the people with whom they are working.

As so often in people-work, there is no single form or words that must be used. Each worker needs to find a way of tackling these issues and a form of words that they feel comfortable with using. The following suggestion is designed to get you thinking.

> Thank you for coming to see me today, J. Before we go any further I need to explain a few things to you about confidentiality. I hope you realise that we will deal with you with the utmost respect and that what you say to us will not go outside this office unless in very exceptional circumstances. One of the ways in which we try to give you the best possible service is to ensure that I as a (student) worker can seek guidance and advice from my manager/supervisor, and this is what I will be doing with the work we will be doing together.
>
> But there will be occasions with some people, J , when they tell us things which we then have to do something about. The sort of thing I mean is when we hear about children or vulnerable adults being abused or put at risk. If we hear about that sort of thing we are legally bound to inform social services or the police, so that they can investigate, and I am sure you appreciate the importance of that. Other than that, J, we would always seek your consent before we spoke to anyone else about you. And even if we felt we had to contact the social services or police we would tell you that that is what we were going to have to do. Now I'm sorry if this sounded a bit long-winded, J, but I hope you understand how important it is.

Exercise 2

Spend some time thinking about the above suggested statement. Re-draft it so that you would feel comfortable about how to explore these issues with your service users. Take this to supervision.

Is there any merit in having an agreed form of words put into writing to give to your service users to take away with them after your meeting?

What about people whose communication skills may need a different approach from you – are there pictorial ways in which this basic information could be put across?

Final thoughts

Confidentiality is one of the core values of all people-work; it will repay some careful attention so that you are completely familiar with what is involved for your agency, and that you are comfortable with how you explain it to your service users.

Further reading

Carnwell, R. and Buchanan, J. (2005) *Effective Practice in Health and Social Care – A Partnership Approach*. Maidenhead: Open University Press.

Hugman, R. (2005) *New Approaches in Ethics for the Caring Professions*. Basingstoke: Palgrave Macmillan.

Trevithick, P. (2005) *Social Work Skills: A Practice Handbook*. 2nd edition. Maidenhead: Open University Press.

Related concepts   establishing a professional relationship; non-verbal communication; partnership working; supervision; whistle blowing.

Conflict Management

Conflict is at the very heart of people-work, especially for professionals such as social workers and probation officers who are often required to balance individual rights and freedoms against risks and harm to others. The very act of undertaking a risk assessment on an individual or family carries with it the likelihood of decisions being taken with which some of the people involved may violently disagree. To remove a child 'at risk' from a family to a place of safety, or to insist that someone in mental distress goes into hospital for treatment, is to be involved in conflict. To develop appropriate communication skills for dealing with conflict, therefore, is essential.

It is worth pausing for a moment to take stock of just how pervasive this theme of conflict is within people-work.

Exercise 1

Jot down as many examples as you can think of where conflict has occurred in your workplace, or in a setting where you have been involved as a student or trainee. Note what the issues were – who was involved – and how it made various people feel? Try also to identify the power issues involved.

Your list will probably be quite a long one, and as this discussion unfolds it will be useful to refer back to it from time to time.

One of the first things to note is that conflict need not necessarily be a bad thing. We have all come across organisations and teams of people who have become comfortable, even complacent, in how they are performing and fulfilling their tasks and roles. If we are honest, most of us prefer 'a quiet life' when we can get on with things in a familiar way, and to have fixed and familiar routines can be of tremendous help when workloads escalate. But best practice, linked to a commitment to incorporating the findings of relevant research into our practice, means that we need to be challenged and stretched, and this is not always a comfortable experience. A new manager may see things in a different light, and new policies and procedures may be introduced specifically to improve the agency's service delivery. In such situations conflict may be seen as a positive experience, as new ways of working come into conflict with older methods within an overall commitment to improve the quality of the services being provided.

Nevertheless, conflict is a complex issue. If you refer to your list from Exercise 1 you may well have included examples of conflict in the following areas:

- you may find yourself 'at odds' with your manager/organisation about the best way of dealing with certain situations
- you may face an internal conflict within yourself over a moral or ethical issue and how you are expected to behave at work – dealing with abortion or drug misuse, for example
- you may vehemently disagree with national or local government policy in an area of work with which you are involved – implementing cuts in services, for example, or how most effectively to supervise serious offenders in the community
- you may 'fall out' with a colleague at work due to a personality clash or difference of opinion
- your team may be split in its opinions about how best to proceed on a certain issue
- you may be called upon to take, or to support, industrial action against your employer
- your service user may have strongly differing opinions about what is the best thing for you both to do when tackling certain problems.

These are a few snapshots of the world of conflict that is at the heart of people-work. In all of them you will no doubt have to take decisions that are difficult, and you certainly will not be able to please all of the people all of the time. But the fact remains that it is not just that decision-taking is difficult – it is also important to practise the communication skills that will be needed to implement them.

As always, core communication skills are essential in such situations. When conflict involves your work with service users or carers, then the following 'golden rules' always apply:

- be open and honest and clear in what you are doing, and explain clearly why you are doing it
- remind people that they have the right not just of reply but of challenging you through appropriate channels
- see people face-to-face, and allow them the opportunity to voice their concerns, however vociferously; ensure that these views are recorded, with a copy given to them for their information.

It is also helpful to have a framework within which to work when handling conflict. This will give you an added confidence in dealing with stressful situations. Thompson (2006) has suggested what he calls the **RED approach** to managing conflict. In this framework **R** stands for **recognising** the conflict. This seems an obvious point to make, but unless the conflict is recognised and named as such, there is a risk that it will not be tackled. We are all familiar with a general sense of unease, or a feeling that all is not quite as it should be, and often we ignore it and hope that it will go away. The act of acknowledging that this is due to a conflict is an important first step towards dealing with it. In his discussion of this point (2006: 114) Thompson also reminds us of the tendency we have to individualise difficulties and to regard the 'other people' as being difficult or uncooperative, whereas the truth may lie elsewhere in a much broader context.

E requires us to **evaluate** the conflict. Few of us wish to be constantly on the lookout for trouble, and one of the skills of our job is to know when to deal with an issue 'head on', and when to leave it well alone. The key point here, however, is the importance of making that decision, and coming to a view about how serious or otherwise the conflict really is. Without doubt, if it is serious and is disregarded, then the chances of it festering and gradually worsening are high. The evaluation of conflict requires us to try to get behind the behaviours and language of the people concerned, and to gain as clear a picture as possible about what the conflict is really about. This will enable us to take the third and final step of **dealing** with it (**D**).

Thompson warns us against the twin dangers of (1) an ostrich-like 'head in the sand' ignoring of the problem altogether, and by contrast (2) an over-reaction which can escalate and exacerbate the difficulties. It is in the *appropriate* dealing with the conflict that the real communication skills lie. In some situations, mediation skills may be useful to help people in dispute work towards a resolution. As a general rule, however, it is important to feel comfortable about taking the risk of asking people what is the matter, or saying that you sense that something is wrong, or wondering if there is anything you can do to help ease the situation. These gentle 'opening' questions or statements may be sufficient to open the lines of communication, and to begin to tease out what the difficulties really are.

Once they become clear, of course, then a further evaluation will be needed to decide what action, if any, is necessary to resolve the problems that have been identified.

Exercise 2

Please re-visit your list of conflict situations from Exercise 1. Choose one or two to work through with your supervisor or practice teacher, and use the RED framework as a way of exploring how to move forward with the scenario(s) you have identified.

Final thoughts

No one pretends that managing conflict is easy or stress-free – exactly the opposite is often the case, although it must also be said that some people seem to thrive on conflict and get a real 'buzz' from it. But if conflict is ignored it is unlikely to go away, and if it festers it is likely to be even harder to handle when the bubble eventually bursts. What you are encouraged to do as a result of reading this entry, therefore, is not to assume that you will need a whole new range of specialised communication skills to deal with conflict. Instead, you are encouraged to be true to yourself, to be honest and open with yourself and others, and to use a framework such as the RED approach to enable you to apply your basic skills to the resolution of conflict.

But do remember – some conflicts can only be handled higher up the chain of command, and that sometimes the only responsible thing to do is to report your concerns to your manager, supervisor or practice teacher, and ask for them to deal with the issues at that level.

References and Further reading

Charlton, R. and Dewdney, M. (2004) *The Mediator's Handbook: Skills and Strategies for Practitioners.* 2nd edition. London: Sweet & Maxwell.

Thompson, N. (2006) *People Problems.* Basingstoke: Palgrave Macmillan.

Stewart, S. (1998) *Conflict Resolution: A Foundation Guide.* Winchester: Waterside Press.

Related concepts Mediation skills; non-verbal communication; reflective practice; supervision.

Counselling

There is a clear overlap between counselling, counselling skills, and people-work in all its great variety, but it is of critical importance that you are clear about the distinctions between them. It is not appropriate to regard counselling as a woolly 'catch-all' activity that is part of every people-worker's tool-kit; but it *is* wholly appropriate to expect all people-workers to use at least some counselling skills in their day-to-day work.

Exercise 1

Spend some time trying to define what you understand counselling to mean. Then see how many different definitions you can find for this complex activity. You might want to undertake a 'Google search' to help you do this. Can you identify common themes? How do these definitions help in clarifying or describing what you do with your service users?

One of the problems you may discover in this search is that counselling is sometimes used in a generalised rather than specific way, sometimes even as a synonym for advice. Students who fail their exams, for example, are often advised to go for academic counselling, by which is meant they need to seek academic guidance and advice about what they did wrong and how they could improve their performance. In-depth exploration of their deepest feelings and aspirations would not be on the agenda for such an encounter.

Feltham and Dryden (1993: 6) produced a definition which has proved popular in the literature. They describe counselling as being:

> A principled relationship characterized by the application of one or more psychological theories and a recognised set of communication skills, modified by experience, intuition and other interpersonal factors, to clients' intimate concerns, problems or aspirations. Its predominant ethos is one of facilitation rather than of advice-giving or coercion. It may be of very brief or long duration, take place in an organisational or private practice setting, and may or may not overlap with practical, medical and other matters of personal welfare.

Counselling is a generic term, and books about it will describe a wide variety of approaches and styles that are now in common practice. Their common theme and purpose is to work with their clients to help them resolve sometimes deep-seated difficulties, clarify their hopes, fears and aspirations, and move into the future in a more positive and dynamic way as a result of this intervention. This is clearly not the job description for any and every people-worker.

Counselling skills again cover a wide range of interventions, from what we may call the 'hard' end (for example, in-depth psychological interviewing) to the 'soft' end of active listening skills, which are the basic building blocks of all communication skills. It is these 'soft end' skills which are the common denominator for all people-work.

Boundaries

You need to be clear in your own mind, in whatever branch of people-work you are involved with, about the boundaries of your skills. This will be the point at which you will need to begin seriously to assess whether the person you are working with needs to be referred to another agency, where perhaps expert counselling help can be made available.

For example, you may be working in a criminal justice setting where you have the responsibility to work with offenders to address and modify their offending behaviour. This will involve using a range of skills and suggesting various strategies for people to use to control, for example, their anger or their abusive behaviour. If, however, a member of the group begins to feel the need to explore a past relationship with an abusive parent, which may have had a significant impact upon his or her current attitudes and behaviour, then this would suggest that a referral to a trained counsellor would be appropriate, alongside (but not instead of) the work you are doing in your group.

Exercise 2

Think about your current role. Where are the boundaries for you and your agency between the generic listening skills and more in-depth work with your service users? Are you clear about how and when you need to refer to other agencies? What are the key agencies in your area who can take these referrals?

Final thoughts

There is a vast literature on counselling if you wish to explore it further. The key point for this book, however, is to identify what are the common skills that every helping professional needs in order to do the job effectively. These are described in this book as active listing skills, and they form the bedrock of the core communication skills that are essential to all people-work.

References and Further reading

Coulshed, V. and Orme, J. (2006) *Social Work Practice*. 4th edition. Basingstoke: Palgrave Macmillan.
Cosis Brown, H. (2002) 'Counselling'. In Adams, R. et al. (2002) *Social Work: Themes, Issues and Critical Debates*. 2nd edition. Maidenhead: Open University Press.
Feltham, C. and Dryden, W. (1993) *Dictionary of Counselling*. London: Whurr.
Miller, L. (2006) *Counselling Skills for Social Work*. London: Sage.
Nelson-Jones, R. (2006) *Theory and Practice of Counselling and Therapy*. 4th edition. London: Sage.

Related concepts Acceptance; active listening; confidentiality; empathy; establishing a professional relationship.

Court Room Skills

Without doubt, appearing in court as a professional people-worker can be daunting even to the experienced; to the inexperienced it can be positively frightening. And yet court work can be a significant part of a people-worker's role, especially if your work involves the criminal justice system or family work. You may be called to court because it is your responsibility to prepare a report for the court on someone who has committed an offence, so that the court can come to a fully informed decision about the most appropriate sentence. You may be involved with a family where separation and divorce mean that expert advice needs to be made available as to what is in the best interests of the child(ren) involved. Or you may go to court to offer a character witness for someone you are working with. Whether you attend court regularly, or it is more of a 'one-off', it is in everyone's best interest that you do as good a job as possible while you are there.

There is no better way of finding out what a court is like than going to see for yourself.

Exercise 1

Make arrangements to go to your local Magistrates' Court As a member of the public you should be allowed to sit in at the back to observe the proceedings. There will be ushers in the entrance area of the court, usually wearing a black gown to make them easily identifiable. Ask them to help you and show you where you can sit. Spend a couple of hours absorbing the atmosphere and getting used to what is happening. That will help you make more sense of the issues we are raising in this discussion. You may of course also want to visit a Crown Court that deals with more serious cases, and where a judge will preside. The system is very similar in that you may sit in the public area, and the ushers will help you to find your way around. If you encounter difficulties, write to the Clerk to the Magistrates, explain why you would like to visit, and you should receive a positive response.

Exercise 2

Undertake some background reading into the English Legal System so that you can understand the basic principles and procedures of the English Legal System. It will also help you understand who does what, and where you might fit into the system if called to attend in your professional role.

Bear in mind too that as a citizen you may be called to undertake jury service at some point in your life. This will give you a very clear picture of how the system works, but not everyone is called to do this, and you will have no idea when the summons for jury service letter will drop onto your door mat!

Some key skills

There are some key skills that are relevant to court work, one of the most of important of which is preparation.

Preparation

General preparation is best undertaken by completing the two intro-ductory exercises suggested above. This will help to orientate you to the context of the court and what is expected of you. In your organisation there should be some more experienced colleagues who can also talk you through what is involved; indeed, you may be able to shadow one of them when they go to court.

Specific preparation becomes necessary when you have a particular reason for going to court. Whether it is a criminal case or a family law matter, it is imperative that you immerse yourself thoroughly in both the detail and the general outline of the case. There may be files you need to read; certainly you will want to meet the person(s) involved and interview them carefully.

Report writing

If you are preparing a report there may be other sources of information you need to tap into, and other professionals whose opinions you may need to canvass. Many organisations will have detailed guidelines as to what a report should contain, and you will be required to complete your report succinctly using the agreed headings. There are three skills you need to develop in your report writing.

First, you need to be succinct. Courts will not want to have to wade through pages and pages of a report: they need information sum-marised for them succinctly, and this is a really important communica-tion skill you need to develop for this kind of work.

Second, you need the skill to be able to separate facts from opinions, and to make this clear in your report. Your professional opinion is certainly val-ued by the court and will be sought, but you need to separate this out from the facts which need to be stated as part of the background and context.

Third, you need the skill to make a recommendation to the court which is legally appropriate, carefully thought through, and which draws, where appropriate, upon relevant research and professional knowledge to make it an informed opinion. Bear in mind, though, that you may well be challenged in court over your report, so you need to be confident about what you are saying.

There is a further skill in how you share your report with the person who is the subject of it. They may or may not agree with some of the things you have said. If there are issues of accuracy then they can help you correct these before the final report is prepared. But often you may be making judgments about them and their behaviour that they may find difficult to accept; they may disagree with the recommendations in the report. This is often the case in divorce cases where one parent may feel that your recommendations about contact and residence are 'not in their favour'. It is helpful, therefore, to spend enough time with the person to tell them what you are proposing in the report, and to explain why you have come to the decisions you have. But you can also tell them that, if they disagree, there are avenues open to them to chal-lenge what you are saying. Their solicitor, of course, is the obvious person to do this for them.

Your skills at communicating with the person over your report also need to take into account their ability to read and understand what you have written. It is far too easy to assume that other people can read, so you need to find sensitive ways of checking this out. Some may find a typewritten court report rather daunting to read, and may ask you to read it to them, especially if the language seems too formal. In all cases, however, it is important to give them an opportunity to ask questions about the report, and to be invited to tell you in their own words what the main themes or recommendations are, so that you can be confident that they have understood what has been said about them.

Your day in court

There are some useful guidelines for the communication skills you will need in court. The non-verbal communication skills you will use, even before you go into the actual court room, include: dressing appropriately; arriving in good time; making sure you contact the right people who are involved; adopting a professional calm and confident manner (even if the butterflies in your tummy are being hyperactive!); and having all the relevant documents and paperwork easily and accessibly available. It is important to seek out the relevant solicitors or barristers to let them know you have arrived; to discuss your report with them, and to gain some idea whether they wish to call you to give evidence. It is helpful to have some advance warning of any issues that they feel need to be expanded on by you, so that you can prepare yourself. You do not always have this luxury, but where possible do ask them if they think the court will require, or benefit from, additional information from you. Not that you should feel constrained by their views: if you feel strongly that you need to speak up in court, then do ask the appropriate solicitor or barrister to call you to the stand.

When you are called into court by the usher, you will have your designated place. If you have taken the opportunity to go to a court for an observational visit, you will be familiar with what is often called the courtroom drama and choreography, which you need to understand in order to know where you fit in. This includes everyone standing when the magistrates (or judge) enter; knowing the order in which the various participants make their contributions, and where you need to go in order to give your evidence. You will be asked for your report by the usher who will ensure that the bench (as the magistrates are sometimes referred to) have copies to read.

When called to present your report in a criminal case, you will be guided by the usher to the witness box where your first responsibility is to take the oath to promise 'to tell the truth, the whole truth and nothing but the truth'. There are various options here. The most common of these is to take the Holy Bible in your right hand and to swear your oath. If you belong to other faith communities, there should be other appropriate holy books for you to use instead of the Bible. However, many people feel unhappy about swearing an oath on a holy book, either because they do not believe in what the holy book represents, or as believers they feel it is not right for them to do this. Therefore it is always possible to make a simple statement or affirmation to the court, promising to tell the truth. Whichever method you choose, the result is the same: you are honour-bound to tell the truth as best you can. To give false information or to seek deliberately to mislead a court are very serious offences, and can be punishable by imprisonment. Your own agency may also take disciplinary action against you if you deliberately seek to mislead the court in any way.

In court proceedings that deal with divorce and family matters, you may find that the whole process is somewhat less formal. You may be called to speak from where you are seated around the table, for example. But the basic rules of behaviour and honesty still apply.

Once in the witness box, you will be asked to confirm your name and your occupation. You may then be asked questions arising from your report. This is the moment when panic may set in; it is also the moment when some basic rules will help you deal with this effectively. These include:

- Take a deep breath and stay looking calm and professional.
- Speak clearly and not too quickly.
- Take your time when answering: it is perfectly acceptable to take a few moments 'thinking time' before you respond to a question.
- State what you know or what you believe, and then stop. If further information is required you will be asked for it.
- Address your comments directly to the magistrates, and remember to refer to them as 'your worship(s)' or at Crown Court, 'your honour'.
- If you are not sure of something, say so. Do not try to cover up your uncertainty with 'off the cuff' comments which have not been thought through.
- If you take your file or notes into the witness box and need to refer to them in order to give an answer, first ask the bench if you may refer to them. Take your time in referring to them, but remember, this is where careful preparation is essential. No one (least of all you) wants to be kept waiting while you struggle to find particular documents in your files.
- Try not to get flustered under cross-examination. Stick to what you have put in the report. By all means give additional information if you have it, but remember that you probably know more about this case than anyone else in the court, except for the person being dealt with. Answer calmly; give your reasons for your opinion, and let the court decide how much weight to give to it. Remember too that it is the job of solicitors or barristers to test out not only the credibility or reliability of the report but also of you the report writer. If they can upset you, or make you flustered, they will have undermined the recommendations you are making. So try to appear calm, even if inside you feel just the opposite.

No one is pretending that this is easy: indeed, confidence comes only with experience and practice. But if you are well prepared, and have done your best in presenting the report, you will be a credible witness whom the court will take seriously. And take comfort that if the magistrates or judge feels that you are being harassed by a solicitor or barrister, they or sometimes the court clerk will often come to your rescue, and admonish the person concerned.

Remember though: it is not personal. People are just doing their jobs, and trying to test the truth, and to do the best for those whom they represent, just as you are.

After the hearing is over

You may well feel emotionally drained. After all, it is natural to feel that in some ways you and your report have been the ones on trial. You may also feel a bit upset if the court did not follow your recommendation when they decided on their sentence or outcome, but again remember that that is their job and their responsibility. Your task was to furnish them with as much relevant information as possible: their task was to make the decisions.

Whatever the outcome, you will want if possible to see the person about whom you prepared the report. They too will most likely be feeling drained, although the outcome will be what affects them most. A post-hearing interview in the cells will feel different from a more relaxed cup of tea in the court canteen, with the person knowing that they can go home. It is, however, important to spend some time going over the outcome with them. In the heat and anxiety of the courtroom drama it is not easy always to remember what is being said; nor are the implications of certain outcomes always fully appreciated. It is good practice, therefore, to talk them through what has been decided, and what must happen next. Ask them to tell you what *they* think has been decided: you can than correct, fine-tune or supplement their response in whatever way you feel is necessary. Often the solicitor or barrister will also want to talk to them and to you to bring matters to a conclusion, and to make sure that everyone understands the outcome fully.

Before you leave, make sure that any further appointments with you are clearly made and recorded, and remember to say goodbye appropriately.

Final thoughts

It is helpful to be able to talk through your time in court with your supervisor, practice teacher, or an experienced colleague, to help you offload any anxieties or negative feelings you may have, and to bring the whole experience into perspective. If, for example, your recommendation was followed by the court, you may be feeling somewhat elated that you have 'won', and may need to be brought back to earth with a reminder of the work that still has to be done with this person. But primarily, the debriefing will help you identify what went well, and ways in which you could improve your performance on future occasions.

Further reading

Brown, H. and Marriott, A. (2005) *ADR: Principles and Practice.* 2nd edition. London: Sweet & Maxwell.

Finch, E. and Fanfinski, S. (2007) *Legal Skills.* Oxford: Oxford University Press.

Hopkins, G. (1998) *Plain English for Social Services: A Guide to Better Communication.* Lyme Regis: Russell House Publishing.

Partington, M. (2006) *Introduction to the English Legal System.* 3rd edition. Oxford: Oxford University Press.

Seymour, C. and Seymour, R. (2007) *Court Room Skills for Social Workers.* Exeter: Learning Matters.

Related concepts   Advocacy; anti-discriminatory practice; conflict management; interpreters; non-verbal communication.

Ecomaps

Ecomaps are similar to genograms in that they are pictorial representations of relationships between people which you can use both as an aid to recording and interpreting information, and also as a direct tool in your work with people.

There is considerable flexibility with how you might use ecomaps. Certainly there is not the same degree of importance in using symbols correctly as there is in the use of genograms. In some ways, as long as it works for you and you know what it means, then that is acceptable, providing of course that if other workers are going to make use of your artwork subsequently the meaning is also clear to them!

Building block 1

The basic building block for an ecomap is an empty circle drawn on a piece of paper, and repeated for as many times as there are people in the relationship network you are seeking to explore and understand. The easiest way is to draw a circle to represent the person with whom you are currently working, and then to think about the other people in that person's life whom they (or you) wish to include in the picture. The crucial idea of the ecomap is that the distance between the central circle/person and other characters is an important indicator. This could be used simply to represent geographical distance between people, so that family members are placed closest to the central character, and people who live at a distance are situated towards the edge of your page. Or the distances on the page could represent the importance of the people in the central character's life, whereby those most important are situated closest to the centre. People who matter less will be placed out towards the margins even if they happen to live in the same household! In other words, with this use of an ecomap, the closer each person is emotionally to the central character, the nearer they are located to the central circle. By contrast, people who are of less significance or importance are located some way out on the edge of the paper. For example, in diagram 1 the ecomap uses physical distances as the key, but in diagram 2 it is emotional distance which is the driver.

The Ecomap in diagram 1 suggests that A is living at home with his parents P and M, and that there are three friends X, Y, and Z who are important in A's life – they could be friends at school perhaps.

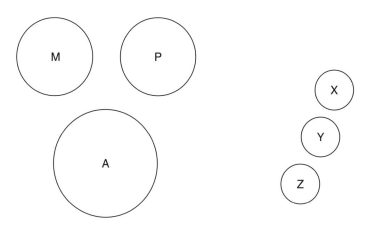

Diagram 1   Physical closeness (provided by Tony Jones)

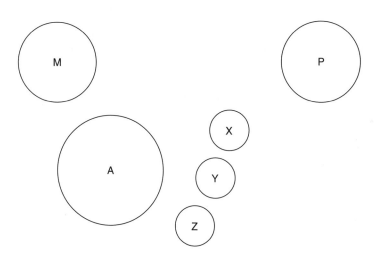

Diagram 2   Emotional closeness (provided by Tony Jones)

The Ecomap in diagram 2 suggests that the people who are emotionally closest to A in the centre are X, Y, and Z, but that crucially P, A's father, although he lives at home with the family, is seen to be distant, and is perceived by A to have a less important influence in A's life.

Building block 2

Into these various circles you can, if you wish or think it is important, write some key information, such as the names, ages, or attributes of each person. If you were working with a young person who was struggling with issues to do with peer pressure, for example, it might be very important to know the ages and characteristics of each of the players who appears on the ecomap, and how these impact upon the person you are working with. The ecomap shown in diagram 2 above would also be enhanced by knowing how old A was – there may be different lessons and implications to be drawn if A was 8, 18 or 28, for example.

Building block 3

In some ways the fun now starts, because at this stage it is possible to use some different symbols to represent the quality of the relationships between the key players. As with the interpretative use of genograms, so with ecomaps, you can use a jagged zig-zaggy line between two people to represent friction, aggression and hostility between them. By contrast, thick strong continuous lines can be used to represent strong relationships between A and those who are most important in A's life, for whatever reason. A thinner line would suggest that the relationship is still important but of lesser significance than the relationship portrayed by the thick line. A dotted line would imply that there is an element of 'take it or leave it' about your relationship to that person.

These observations demonstrate how simple and straightforward the use of ecomaps can be, but also how effectively in just a simple picture a very powerful story can be depicted.

Exercise 1

This is probably a good point at which to pause and invite you to 'have a go' for yourself to see how ecomaps can work. As with any tool which we select to enhance our practice with people, we need to be confident about why we are using it, and what benefits it can bring to our work, and also what risks we may run if we do use it directly with people.

As a starter, draw an ecomap of your life and your relationships using geographical distance as the driver. This means that you will draw a circle for each person who lives with you in the same household

(Continued)

(Continued)

in close proximity to the circle you have drawn to represent yourself. Other people who are important to you, but who live at varying distances from where you live, can be placed on your ecomap at appropriate distances from you.

When you have completed the location of all the people you wish to include, then think about your actual relationship with them, and use a combination of strong lines, weak lines, dotted lines and jagged lines to represent how you feel about your relationship with them.

Exercise 2

This time we will use the idea of emotional significance as the driver for your ecomap. This means that with your own circle again centrally placed on the page, you draw circles close to you representing the people who mean most to you, and place out towards the end of the paper those who matter least to you, depending upon how distant you feel from them emotionally. Put names in each circle so that they become real to you for this exercise.

As with Exercise 1 it is again useful to draw in the relationship lines on the ecomap to indicate clearly which relationships are most nurturing and which are most stressful.

A note of caution

It will have become clear to you in completing these exercises that this deceptively easy tool can be immensely powerful. If you take seriously the issues that it raises, especially in relation to stressful relationships, you can very quickly find yourself in touch with some powerful, even disturbing feelings. This should be a warning to you, therefore, to handle such tools with care, and to regard them as just that: tools to be used, but with caution. It is one thing to use this tool as a way of recording information after an interview and to reflect on the issues that are raised. It is another matter when you begin to use ecomaps in direct work with people. If, therefore, you find yourself getting into difficult territory, it is important to use the same degree of sensitivity as always, and to have the courage to put the tool to one side if need be. There is no particular merit in pressing on in a mechanistic way just to gather information at a surface level, and certainly no justification for pressing on into territory which the person you are working with would find too distressing to handle.

Building block 4 – Fingers on the buttons

So far we have talked about how you can use ecomaps as a pen and paper/flip chart and marker pen exercise, and we have seen how effective and powerful this can be. There is another variation that deserves mention, not least because it can be used with young people and with people who have mild communication difficulties. This variation uses a tin of buttons instead of pen and paper.

You need to have a fairly large tin with a variety of shapes, colours and sizes of buttons. This approach is very much for direct working with people, and has the merit of being interactive. In essence, it is a dynamic ecomap.

After an appropriate introduction as to why this tool is being used, the person with whom you are working is invited to choose a button from the tin that best represents who they are. They put this in the middle of the table – perhaps with an invitation from you to say why that particular button appeals to them and why they have chosen it. Then you go one by one through the people who are important in that person's life, and you ask them to choose a button to represent each of them in turn. Then they are asked to place that button somewhere in the table to present how close they feel to that person. After a while you will end up with several different buttons on the table representing the various people in that person's life. You then have the opportunity to ask about each of them (or you could do this as each button is placed in position).

Again this can be very powerful as the picture unfolds, and sometimes the feelings which are evoked are strongly expressed. On occasion, if you wanted to use this tool further, you could move a particular button closer, or further away, from the central button and explore how that would feel to the person with whom you are working.

Final thoughts

As with many tools which can be used to enhance communication skills, ecomaps can be powerful visual representations of complex and at times distressing realities about people's relationships. They can also represent strengths, support systems and networks, and ways in which people's resilience can be enhanced. It is up to you as a worker to decide how most effectively to use such tools, and what themes and issues you feel need to be explored further.

But there is also a warning to be sounded here: however much you may feel you wish to be in charge, it is important to stress that tools like ecomaps are powerful *precisely because* they put the person with whom you are working into the driving seat. Ecomaps can be excellent tools for real partnership-working. It will be up to you, therefore, to listen attentively, so that what you begin really to focus on is what is important to that person, and not what you find easiest to handle.

Further reading

Coulshed, V. and Orme, J. (2006) *Social Work Practice*. 4th edition. Basingstoke: Palgrave Macmillan.
Thompson, N. (2006) *People Problems*. Basingstoke: Palgrave Macmillan.
www.smartdraw.com

Related concepts Assessment; genograms; empowerment; partnership working.

Empathy

Within a wide range of people-work, empathy is a key buzz word, which characterises a high quality relationship between the worker and the person being listened to or helped. Several metaphors have been used to try to capture the essence of empathy, one of the most popular being that of 'wearing another person's shoes or moccasins'. The idea behind this is a simple one: empathy is about trying to see the world from the other person's point of view; to get inside how the other person really feels, so that you can begin to see things through their eyes. Only then will that person feel that they have been accepted and fully listened to.

A distinction is sometimes drawn between sympathy and empathy. We can all feel sympathy towards someone who is going through a difficult time, and we express this by saying how sorry we are, and offering to do anything we can to help. Sympathy is an emotion or feeling that is generated within us by the misfortune of others, and in that sense is part of what it means to be genuinely and fully human. The world would be a poorer place if we were not moved by tragedy and misfortune to offer a variety of responses to others. Indeed much charitable work, on an individual and corporate level, is a channelling of these sympathetic responses in practical, as well as emotional, ways.

Empathy in some ways builds upon this sympathetic streak within us, but seeks to develop a far more interactive relationship with the other person. It is, of course, impossible fully to 'get inside another person's skin' (another metaphor sometimes used), but the attempt to do so is hugely important within a professional relationship. It is only when the other person begins to feel that you really do understand 'where they are coming from', and can glimpse the world from their point of view, that they will begin to feel accepted, and encouraged to begin a journey towards whatever changes in their lives are necessary.

It is in this sense that empathy can be regarded as a communication skill that needs to be recognised, practised and developed. Perhaps it is not a skill in the strict sense of the word: perhaps it says more about the outcome of other communication skills being used effectively. Nevertheless, it is an outcome that a skilled helper can achieve within a professional relationship, without leaving it to chance.

Koprowska (2005: 49) captures the challenge of empathic listening when she talks about 'empathic attunement', which carries the notion of someone trying to tune into a particular radio wavelength to listen to a particular programme. The signals are out there, but it needs some careful and sensitive work on the part of the person adjusting the tuner to 'home in' on the signal so that it is loud and clear. The skill lies in that careful and sensitive adjustment to hear the other person's programme with maximum clarity.

The development of empathic skills is an issue that has taxed trainers and educators alike. Controlled outcome studies by Nerdrum and Lundquist (1995), and Nerdrum (1997) explored the effectiveness of communication skills training in increasing students' capacity to be empathetic. There was sufficient evidence from these studies to argue for these skills to be included in basic communication skills training courses, in spite of other studies which were more sceptical (e.g., Barber, 1988). There is also a wider concern about how students are able to transfer the skills gained in the training context into their eventual professional practice (Dickson and Bamford, 1995). Although this remains a largely under-researched issue, the implications from these findings are clear: there is no automatic achievement of empathetic attunement, and workers need to put every effort into achieving this goal with those with whom they are professionally engaged.

The following suggestions may help you to develop your skills in this area. They are based on guidelines that have been drawn up by tutors at the University of Manchester involved in training medical students in communication skills, but are applicable to a wide range of people-workers. They are not foolproof, and must always be used with sensitivity, but if used well, they can help you build up an empathic rapport with the person with whom you are working.

- Acknowledge verbal cues: e.g., you have just told me how sad you feel when ...
- Acknowledge non-verbal cues: e.g., you seem to me to be very tense/angry/upset.
- Use tentative questions: e.g., I'm wondering whether you feel this way because of ...
- Use of self-disclosure: e.g., I think that if that were me I would feel very shocked/upset by what you have just described to me.
- Use your imagination: e.g., I imagine you must have felt very ....
- Gentle touch: e.g., reaching out gently to touch the person's hand, arm or shoulder can sometimes be a powerful expression of empathic attunement, but obviously it needs to be carefully considered especially across gender or cultural boundaries. If in doubt, it is better not to risk it, but you will be surprised at how even a slight movement of the hand towards the other person can be equally effective.
- Use mirroring: e.g., adjust your tone of voice, posture and gestures to mirror those of the other person. This can convey a strong rapport, but can also be rather off-putting if done mechanistically. Sometimes, however, if the other person is sitting in a very enclosed posture with arms folded, etc., you can begin by mirroring that posture, and slowly but deliberately open up your own posture to encourage them to follow.

Exercise 1

To complete this exercise you will need to have someone to discuss some examples from your work, and who can help you explore your effectiveness at developing empathy. Your supervisor, line manager or practice teacher should be able to help, but it is important that you can trust them to work with you at a fairly deep level. In a word, you need to be confident that they can establish an empathic relationship with you.

(Continued)

(Continued)

Choose an interview you have recently completed, and review it with regard to the communication skills you used. How successfully do you feel you were in establishing empathic rapport with this person? What were the issues you struggled with in 'tuning in' to them? How would you put into words the world-view which they held, and how clearly do you feel you were able to acknowledge and explore it with them? How might you have conducted the interview differently to achieve a stronger rapport with them?

Final thoughts

Getting inside someone else's world-view is one of the main themes of the contemporary debate about spirituality, with its interest in 'what makes people tick', how they view the world, and what gives people meaning and purpose in their lives. As we engage with people at this deeper level that is the goal of empathic attunement, we may begin to understand the deeper relevance of this theme of spirituality to our work with other people.

References and Further reading

Barber, J. (1988) 'Are microskills worth teaching?', *Journal of Social Work Education*, Winter, no.1: 3–12.

Dickson, D. and Bamford, D. (1995) 'Improving the interpersonal skills of social work students: the problem of transfer of training and what to do about it', *British Journal of Social Work*, 25: 85–105.

Kopsrowska, J. (2005) *Communication and Interpersonal Skills in Social Work*. Exeter: Learning Matters.

Miller, J. (2006) *Counselling skills for Social Work* London: Sage.

Nerdrum, P. and Lundquist, K. (1995) 'Does participation in communication skills training increase student levels of communicated empathy? A controlled outcome study', *Journal of Teaching in Social Work*, 12: 139–156.

Nerdrum, P. (1997) 'Maintenance of the effect of training in communication skills: a controlled follow-up study of level of communicated empathy', *British Journal of Social Work*, 27: 705–722.

Trevithick, P. (2005) *Social Work Skills – A Practice Handbook*. Maidenhead: Open University Press. (p. 153 ff)

Related concepts Active listening; establishing a professional relationship; feedback; non-verbal communication; reflective practice; spirituality.

Empowerment, Resilience and a Strengths Perspective

We are dealing here with a clutch of inter-related concepts, all of which are effectively dealt with at length certainly in the professional social work literature, but which, from a communication skills perspective, can usefully be viewed together. They all deal with the impact which we hope our intervention skills will have: from being perhaps disempowered, helpless and overwhelmed, we hope that they will emerge at the end of the helping process feeling much better able and equipped to cope, feeling much more in control of their lives and in touch with powers of resilience and inner strengths of which, under the pressures of their problems, they had temporarily lost sight.

As with other issues we are discussing, there is a clear overlap of values and skills. In this instance, there is a responsibility upon all people-workers to examine their value-base, and how this informs their view of the people who come to them for help. We can be sure that how we feel about other people will come across in our non-verbal communication. If, for example, we view our service users or clients as people without hope, vision or 'moral fibre', or as 'inadequate', 'incapable', 'misfits', 'deviants', or 'scroungers', it will be almost impossible to disguise these value judgments in the way we deal with them. People will quickly get the message that that is how we regard them. And the question has then to be asked, is this how we would like to be treated if the tables were turned?

The likelihood is that we ourselves would not wish to be treated or regarded in such a way: we would regard it as being insulting, degrading and demeaning. And then it dawns on us that we have fallen prey to the trap of professional pride, in which the world falls into two groups: the helpers and the helped. We the helpers are basically OK: we are competent and deserving of respect; on the other hand those who need to be helped are somehow second-class citizens to be pitied; they may be offered a helping hand, but somehow they are of less worth than the rest of us.

This stark juxtaposition of viewpoints is intended to highlight the power of value judgments, and the ways in which they can obstruct best anti-discriminatory practice. It also is intended to reveal the falseness of such an approach. Unless you work from a value-base that accords dignity and respect to each and every other human being, no matter what their circumstances, you are running the risk of developing this two-tier mentality which can be so destructive of good people-work.

It will be quite different, of course, if your value-base reflects an alternative approach. If you view other people as having the capacity for good as well as evil; as having latent strengths as well as inherent weaknesses; as having the potential for taking control over their lives even in the most difficult of circumstances, then this approach will communicate itself to them in both subtle and direct ways in how you work with them. At a very profound level this is at the heart of all communication skills in people-work.

How you go about achieving this is the big challenge, although by now it should be clear that the first, and biggest, step is clarifying your own mind-map and how you regard those who come to you for help. From the basic stance of according dignity, respect and acceptance to each person, there flows a set of communication skills that you will need to cultivate and develop. These include:

Acceptance   The basic communication skill of demonstrating to another person that you accept them, 'warts and all', is a fundamental starting point for all empowerment.

Explaining   This is a relatively simple skill to use, and people-workers sometimes overlook how helpful and liberating it can be for people to be offered explanations. Sometimes, when we are feeling overwhelmed, we can't see things clearly: we talk about 'not being able to see the wood for the trees', and what we often need is for someone to explain things to us. Classic examples of this are official communications from people in authority. It does not seem to matter that every effort has been made by them to write to us in clear, plain English; in the heat of the moment people can panic, and assume the worst. Sometimes, therefore, the role of the people-worker is to read such communications carefully, and to explain what is being said 'in words of one syllable'. On occasion, the letter may well make people feel that the worst is imminent – that they are going to be evicted, or have their electricity cut off, or their benefit payments stopped. In such cases there may be appeal procedures that can be explained, or additional sources of help and advice that can be called upon. Such explanations can be hugely important.

Another area where explanations can be helpful is in interpreting and explaining other people's behaviour. Parents often become distressed with how their children are behaving; older people worry about the loss of various skills and faculties; members of minority groups may not always appreciate that the law is there to protect them against oppression and abuse. While there are no simplistic answers, sometimes an explanation, based on accurate knowledge and relevant research findings, can be very reassuring and supportive.

You should also not underestimate the importance of explaining what the law says, and what can be done legally to challenge certain decisions or actions. Some people, for example, value information about various pressure groups that exist to challenge aspects of social injustice, and welcome explanations about how they operate in the local and wider community.

Finally, it is becoming increasingly liberating to explain to people what information is available to them electronically, via the Internet and through the websites of a wide variety of organisations. The information explosion is both liberating and bewildering, and sometimes it is the role of the people-worker to explain to people which sources of information are most useful, reputable and bona fide. It is, of course, dangerous to assume computer literacy, just as it is unwise to assume that everyone can read and write. So any explanations about the availability of electronic information needs to be tempered with a sensitive exploration about whether the person is able to access this information easily, or whether they would welcome being put in touch with a local organisation that can help them achieve this.

Exercise 1

Consider your own agency and the work you do. What are the key sources of information that are of most use and benefit to those who come to you. How do you make these available to people? What can you do to make these resources more accessible?

Encouraging   It is a truism to say that everyone needs encouragement, but in people-work it is particularly important to find and develop ways of encouraging people that do not come across as patronising, unrealistic or shallow. It is easy to overlook people's strengths and resilience when they come to see you and are overwhelmed by a particular set of difficulties. People-workers tend to get used to people who seem dis-empowered and unable to complete some mutually agreed tasks that were agreed at their previous meeting. It is tempting then to take over, and to begin to do things for people: it is often quicker, but in the long run it is counter-productive. Significantly, it risks undermining what self-confidence the person still has.

To be encouraging of others, therefore, is a key communication skill in people-work, both among colleagues and with those who come to us for help. Try to find at least two things in each encounter or interview which merit a word of encouragement: this will be a huge motivation for future progress.

The words to use must be chosen with care, of course. A glib, hearty 'well done' may be extremely patronising, and people will often know deep down whether or not they have given their 'best shot' at a particular task or undertaking. Nevertheless, to say 'well done' at an appropriate point can be greatly appreciated, as can other forms of encouragement. For example:

> J, this is really good – I know you feel you struggle at times, but I think you've done really well doing this.

> Not many people would have been able to do this, J.

> I know you must feel disappointed at not having done as well as we had hoped, but well done for having a stab at it – it would have been easy to throw in the towel.

> J, to have done this on top of everything else you have been worrying about is really good – you can feel proud of yourself.

Asking   There are several ways in which sensitive questioning or asking can be an empowering experience. Sometimes this may involve stepping outside the immediate 'circle of distress' and asking some more general focused questions that can 'take the heat out of things' by trying to put the other person in touch with their strengths and resilience. It also helps you gain a fuller, better picture of the whole person, not just the presenting problems. For example:

- Ask people about what they are good at, and how they would normally handle a difficulty. This may produce a response that demonstrates their strengths, but which also highlights the particularly disabling features of this problem that has temporarily got the better of them.
- Ask them what they feel good about themselves, their life or their family, or what they enjoy most. This again may help them get back in touch with positive aspects of their lives that have temporarily been blotted out by their current problems. This has to be done sensitively of course: they may feel that there is nothing to report. You may need therefore to be gently persistent, but this is worth doing because it reinforces the value-base of all people-work that you are seeking to communicate to them, that each individual is of value,

worth and importance, and has inner gifts, strengths and the inner potential and capacity to cope, albeit with the help of other people from time to time.

• You can also gently ask questions about who has told the person in some way or other that they are not capable of dealing with difficulties. This is territory that can trespass into counselling and therapeutic interventions, which are not the domain of all people-work of course, so sensitivity is called for in exploring this theme. Nevertheless, in a low-key way, this question may be very revealing. People may begin to think back and reflect upon how their parents, or a teacher at school, or close friends, relatives or partners have 'put them down' and given them the message that they are 'no good'. This then provides you with an opportunity to challenge that perception, and to ask them whether they wish to continue to live under its domination, or to reassert themselves, to break out and take more control over their lives and actions. In some cases, of course, you may feel that a referral to a counsellor may be a very creative step for the person to take to 'kick-start' their personal journey towards liberation from these disempowering influences.

Task sharing   There is a strong emphasis in people-work on the importance of partnership-working and task-sharing. This is for a very good reason. If as people-workers we simply take over and do things *for* or even *to* the other person, however well meaning it may be, this risks undermining the capacity and confidence of the other person, and begins to inculcate a spirit of dependency upon the worker. Task-sharing counteracts that risk by insisting from the outset that a pattern and a programme of shared tasks is negotiated by them both.

The notion of a programme is important here. There are some situations where the person in need is so distressed and disempowered that the worker has to take responsibility for the first step of the journey. This may be, for example, contacting the housing department over an eviction order, or a debt company to begin the process of review and repayment and putting everything 'on hold'. Similarly, someone with acute mental health difficulties that requires immediate hospital treatment, will need the professionals to take responsibility to ensure that diagnosis and treatment are put into immediate effect. If there are overriding concerns about the protection of vulnerable children or adults, then steps must be taken without delay to ensure their safety. Someone seriously under the influence of alcohol or drugs may need steps to be taken to ensure their safety until they return to a level of sobriety where they can begin to take serious responsibility for their future. The concept of a programme, therefore, is important because it needs to include the possibility of a worker having to act quickly and decisively, sometimes with the other person's consent, sometimes without it. At a later stage, however, the tasks will be more evenly shared, and towards the end it will be the worker who sits back because the other person will have gained sufficient self-confidence and resilience to take the lead and become more independent.

As the situation unfolds, therefore, the worker will want to begin to explore ways of sharing tasks in order to facilitate and empower the other person to take responsibility for their lives. The person whose lifestyle has become chaotic, resulting, for instance, in the non-payment of bills, will need to decide whether this is a downwards spiral from which they are desparate to escape. If that is so, then they will need to begin taking some responsibility for taking steps to achieve this, with the support of the worker. If they do not wish to escape, then there is little the worker can do apart from some immediate 'firefighting', because the situation will keep on recurring. People whose behaviour puts others at risk will need to begin to take responsibility for the consequences of their actions, and to decide whether or not they wish to change this cycle of disruption. If they do, then the worker can begin exploring parenting classes, offending behaviour sessions, or anger management courses in which the person concerned begins to re-take control over their life to develop a more creative lifestyle which does not damage others. The person under the influence of drugs or alcohol similarly needs to take decisions about who or what is in control of their lives. It is not a decision that anyone else can take for them, but there are people who can share their journey with support and encouragement and skilled interventions.

The skill with task-sharing comes in the negotiation and staging of the tasks which are to be mutually agreed. Too much, too soon can be daunting and disabling; too little can be demeaning and off-putting. It is always important, therefore, to check with the person how they feel about the tasks that are being negotiated, and their capacity to deal with them. And when they report back it is crucial to praise what has been accomplished even if it is somewhat less than had been hoped for, and not to let setbacks be anything other than temporary. In fact setbacks can be very enlightening because they throw up issues which perhaps had not been fully thought through beforehand when the tasks were being negotiated. An exploration into exactly why this task could not be fully completed may be very revealing for everyone concerned.

Implicit in all of this, of course, is the commitment you need to have to task-sharing. You need to be clear what you will be doing to help move things forward, and to ensure that you 'deliver the goods' by doing what you say you will do. But do also ensure that this process does not become competitive or point-scoring: it is all part of a restorative process to enable the other person to manage perfectly well without you.

Exercise 2

Think about some of the people with whom you have been or still are working. Where on the spectrum of independency and dependency do you think they are located? In what ways have you negotiated task-sharing? How far have you a clear picture of the programme you need to implement in order for the other person to become fully empowered and able to take full responsibility for their future?

Final thoughts

This section has dealt with important themes that lie at the heart of good communication skills – or rather, good communication skills lie at the heart of these important themes. It is all too easy to convey subtle messages of disapproval, and to invite a comparison between your success, and the other person's failure to deal with life effectively. The communication skills necessary to foster the spirit of empowerment, and to tap into a person's resilience, are a mixture of the 'soft' skills of your attitude towards others and the value-base you seek to embody, and the focused skills of active listening, interviewing and intervention techniques that can help you achieve your mutually agreed objectives. Everyone needs encouragement, and there can be few more rewarding situations than seeing someone regain confidence, resilience and the capacity to lead creative, independent and fulfilled lives.

All this talk about our capacity to facilitate others is based on the assumption that we as workers are flexible, well-supported, and sufficiently in tune with ourselves that we are able to respond to others in creative and effective ways. Pressures of work, however, linked with personal difficulties than can beset all of us from time to time, mean that there will be occasions where our own resilience is undermined and our work with others impaired. Warning signs of these developments must be taken seriously. We need to take care of ourselves if we are ever to be of any use to others. Supervision is meant to be a vehicle for exploring these areas of difficulty, and we owe it to ourselves, our agency and to those we seek to help to ensure that supervision meets our needs.

Further reading

Carnwell, R. and Buchanan, J. (2005) *Effective Practice in Health and Social Care: A Partnership Approach*. Maidenhead: Open University Press.

Harrison, R. et al. (2003) *Partnership Made Painless – A Joined-Up Guide to Working Together*. Lyme Regis: Russell House Publishing.

Marsh, P. and Doel, M. (2005) *The Task-Centred Book*. London: Routledge/Community Care.

Trevithick, P. (2005) *Social Work Skills – A Practice Handbook*. 2nd edition. Maidenhead: Open University Press.

Related concepts   Acceptance; active listening; anti-discriminatory practice; confidentiality; counselling; feedback; non-verbal communication; spirituality; supervision.

Endings

Best practice in people-work means keeping the ending of the professional relationship clearly in mind from the outset. This ensures that clear objectives are set, and that progress towards achieving them is clearly monitored and evaluated. It also ensures that once you have achieved your objectives you will be able to disengage, acknowledge what has been achieved, and say goodbye.

Endings are also important to consider with each and every meeting or interview you hold with the other person, so that the allotted time is used effectively. There is nothing worse than a worker giving implicit or explicit permission to someone to go into 'deep water', which may result in the person getting very upset as they try to make sense of painful experiences, only to be informed a few moments later that 'time is up' and they have to leave. There is then no time for them to regain their composure and return to their everyday world.

In both aspects of endings, there are important communication skills necessary: if they are practised well, the endings can be positive; if they are handled badly, endings can be upsetting and negative experiences.

Exercise 1

Think about some of the endings you have experienced in your life – they may be large-scale events or relatively minor. What do you think makes the difference between a good ending and a poor ending?

This exercise focuses upon your experiences of endings, not least because in people-work our own experiences often colour our approach to practice. How often have we heard people say that they do not like 'goodbyes'; they will do anything to avoid those moments of 'closure'. For whatever reason, they are too painful, and perhaps stimulate within them some personal painful experiences of endings that they do not want to revisit. In saying this, we are not trying to pathologise some people's reluctance to engage with endings, but we are suggesting that, in this area, our own experiences may be a factor in how we deal with other, including professional, endings.

For some people, of course, it is the large-scale events that have cast their shadow. Experiences of tragedy and bereavement, for example, are losses on a grand scale that can seriously influence other less traumatic goodbyes. Like a spilled bottle of ink, their impact seeps into all sorts of hidden corners, so that even faint reminders of the pain are enough to make them 'fight shy' of other types of farewell.

This reinforces the importance of becoming a reflective practitioner. The situations we find difficult to handle, what scares us or makes us feel insecure, these aspects of our personality are not magically left outside the door of the interview room. They come with us, and the secret of good reflective and self-aware practice is not to pretend that they don't exist, but rather to face them and to ensure that they do not encroach on our professional dealings with others. This means that we have an obligation to ourselves, as well as to those whom we seek to help, to explore these issues within supervision so that we can assess their impact upon our practice.

Again, for some people, this whole area of endings and goodbyes raises issues of 'existential angst', which is a rather grandiose, almost pompous way of talking about what sense of meaning and purpose people find in their lives. Thompson (2006: 8) captures this well when he talks of:

> the type of challenges we face simply by being humans, by being in the world and seeking to make sense of it. Existential challenges can generally be seen as crises or turning points in our lives...

These issues of meaning and purpose in our lives are part of the contemporary debate about spirituality, and form the backdrop to this issue of endings. Again, we are not for a moment suggesting that as people-workers we find ourselves wracked with angst at each and every ending we have to deal with. That would be farcical and demeaning to our professional competence. But it does suggest that from time to time certain types of ending will 'get to us', and that this will often tell us more about ourselves than the person with whom we are working.

This discussion takes us back to the importance of non-verbal communication; it is very easy to convey a set of negative messages about endings by our attitude towards them. But it is important that we make every effort to ensure that endings are positive for the people with whom we work, as well as for us as workers. Some useful guidelines for achieving this include:

- Be clear from the outset why you are meeting together, what you need to achieve, and how long this is likely to take.
- Keep your progress regularly under review so that you know how well you are doing and how near you are to completing your tasks.
- Be keen to offer praise to the other person for the progress they are making to help foster their resilience and independence.
- Do not be discouraged by setbacks – few people get it right first time, and there are things to learn from setbacks to help reach the ultimate destination.
- Remind yourself and the other person how much time you have left – this applies both to an individual interview (e.g., 'we only have 15 minutes left today – what do you think we can most usefully do in that time?'), and to the period of time set aside to achieve certain tasks (e.g., 'we agreed we would meet six times; today we are on session 4 – shall we review where we have reached and decide how best to use the remaining two sessions?').
- Allow some time at the end of each interview for the other person to regain their equilibrium if they have been upset; attempt to normalise their re-entry back into their everyday life by asking a couple of ordinary questions about what they are doing for the rest of the day or week, and check that they are feeling OK.
- At the end, spend time acknowledging the achievements and the progress made; affirm the other person's growing independence and capacity to cope; spend some time identifying how the person will cope in the future, and what other tasks may need to be dealt with some way or another.
- End the final session by wishing them well, and saying goodbye properly.
- Finally, write up your records, noting what has been achieved, and how the 'case' has been concluded, so that anyone needing to find out about it in future will have a good accurate record.

Final thoughts

It is often said that 'everyone likes a happy ending', but in your work with people that sounds a somewhat utopian aspiration. Nevertheless, your work should always have a purpose that is clearly defined and time limited, and if you make sure that you achieve at least a satisfactory ending to it, it will give a clear message that it is time for everyone involved to move on.

References and Further reading

Kadushin, A. (1997) *The Social Work Interview: A Guide for Human Service Professionals*. 4th edition. New York: Columbia University Press.

Thompson, N. (2003) *Communication and Language – A Handbook of Theory and Practice*. Basingstoke: Palgrave Macmillan.

Thompson, N. (2006) *People Problems*. Basingstoke: Palgrave Macmillan.

Trevithick, P. (2005) *Social Work Skills: A Practice Handbook*. Maidenhead: Open University Press.

Related concepts   Establishing a professional relationship; loss; non-verbal communication; reflective practice; spirituality.

Establishing a Professional Relationship

It is often said that in people-work of various kinds all that we really have to offer to someone else is ourselves: our toolkit, if you like, is how we relate to the person who comes to us – in short – our communication skills. Whereas a car mechanic would be lost without a box of spanners and an electronic diagnostic machine, and a dentist without the range of drills, 'prodders' and fillings, people-workers are only effective when they have developed the skills to work with the other person in a professional human way.

This is very much a communication skill in its own right, and includes a range of non-verbal communication skills. Perhaps one way of helping to clarify what is meant here is by stating what a professional relationship is *not*.

Exercise 1

Spend some time jotting down what you think should not be part of a professional relationship. Keep these notes beside you as you work through this topic.

As a professional people-worker you are *not*:

- A friend to the other person. You will seek to be friendly towards them, but a friend often offers a far more comprehensive relationship than you can.
- Always and instantly available. You have responsibilities to other service users or clients, as well as to other aspects of your organisation's work. You may sometimes decide to 'drop everything' to respond to a particular crisis with someone, but normally you will work with a system of mutually agreed appointments.
- Offering general 'chat' sessions. There will always be a clear reason for meeting in the first place; a clear set of objectives to work towards, and a clear understanding of when the relationship needs to end.
- Offering an open-ended relationship. Your time with the person will be focused on agreed areas of work, and for an agreed length of time. In fact, in most cases, the end of the relationship will be in sight at the beginning.
- Physically close to the other person. We are much more aware these days of the difficult and at times compromising risks of physical contact between people-workers and those with whom they are seeking to help. Physical contact can be misunderstood; or people can be exploited when a sexual relationship develops between the worker and the other person. However mutually acceptable this may seem at the time, in fact it always constitutes a breach of the boundary of the professional relationship, and therefore is always wrong.

This review of what a professional relationship is *not* is a helpful mirror-image to clarify what you do need to be aiming for when developing this with another person.

The most important aspects of establishing a professional relationship, therefore, are as follows:

- Always be clear yourself and with the other person about why you are meeting and what you need to achieve.
- Always establish clear boundaries, so that each of you knows what is and is not acceptable.
- Always be clear that you are representing your agency, and that you are accountable to your manager for the work you do; explain that this may sometimes involve another colleague sharing in the work with you, or doing something on your behalf, or working with the person instead of you.
- Always be clear that the reward you will receive for your work will be in terms of satisfaction of a job well done. Receiving gifts from grateful service users should normally be tactfully declined – offers of money must always be refused.

  Sometimes, however, you may feel that to refuse a modest gift of appreciation, such as a bunch of flowers or a small box of chocolates, would cause unnecessary hurt. This is a matter of professional judgment, of course, but if you do decide to accept, say that you will take the gift back to your office for other colleagues also to enjoy. On your return, make a written note on the file and copy it to your manager explaining what has been given to you, and that this has been left at the office for general, rather than your own personal enjoyment. Do check with your manager, however, about the team or agency policy on such matters, as this can avoid embarrassment or more serious repercussions (e.g., allegations of accepting bribes).

The problem of transference

You will also need to be aware of at least some psychological aspects of professional relationships. Whereas it is true that a judicious use of ourselves can prove to be highly supportive, encouraging and even therapeutic for those with whom we work, there is a darker side of which you need to be aware. When you become involved professionally with someone else, you never know what memories may be stirred up in the other person – or, for that matter, within yourself. How many times have we said, in our everyday transactions, 'oh, you remind me of so and so', or, 'you are just like ...', or, 'you sound just like...'. For all our uniqueness as individuals, there are some common traits and characteristics, and we all from time to time see other people in the face, voice, body language or behaviour of the person in front of us.

Most of the time we deal with this without any difficulty – we see the 'connection' but then dismiss it, and refuse to let it cloud our dealings with the other person. But not always. The psychological phenomenon called 'transference' is familiar to counsellors and psychoanalysts who work in-depth with people, and who sometimes find that their clients transfer onto them a range of deep-seated feelings, anxieties and needs. These can span a range of emotions from love to hate, and the worker has to be skilled at recognising when this is happening.

Within the more general spheres of people-work, such in-depth work is not part of the role, but nevertheless some degree of transference can still take place. As a worker you may trigger some reaction within the person you are professionally involved with, not because of who you are, how you behave, what you say or how you look, but because something about you stimulates a memory within the other person, and they begin to respond to you as if you were that other person. Or they may begin to hope that you will be able to meet a deeper set of needs than is appropriate to your professional relationship.

Part of your professional response, therefore, will be to recognise that it is not *you as you* that the person is getting very angry about – it is someone else in their past who has caused them hurt which has not been resolved. It is not you they are falling in love with, but someone, or even some imaginary, fantasy person, who they hope will meet their deepest unmet needs. It is not you who makes them react to you as if you were an authoritarian parent; it is some parental figure in the past whose influence is still strongly at work at some deep level in their lives.

When we say, however, that it is not you doing this to them, that is only partially true. There is, of course, something about you that triggers this reaction in them, and you need to be reflecting and asking yourself what this might be. But you need to remain outside this reaction, and not to get drawn into it personally. If you are wise and perceptive, you will be able to work with these feelings and reactions to help the other person begin to understand them, and deal with them more effectively. You will realise that, in these situations, you are being given an insight into some aspects of what makes the other person 'tick', and this may help you gently to tease out whether this sort of reaction to other people is common. If they can begin to see that transference is taking place, it may help them form more effective relationships in future.

There is also, of course, another problem; and that is when someone we are working with triggers off some unexpected and powerful feelings *within us*, and we may find ourselves projecting onto the other person something deep-seated within ourselves. This is where self-awareness is crucial, linked to a supportive, perceptive supervisory relationship where such issues can be sensitively explored, and you can be set free to become a more effective worker. Often it is enough to realise, and to record, that some level of transference is taking place. To see it is to be able to stop it; it does not imply you need in-depth counselling or psychoanalysis to sort it out. Just occasionally, however, the deep waters of your innermost self may be stirred and disturbed by such encounters, and you may then need to seek professional help.

Recording and supervision are important tools in helping you to recognise and deal with transference, both when it occurs in the other person and when it occurs within you. You may feel that a particular interview 'got stuck' for some reason, or that the other person's behaviour or reaction to you was a bit 'skewed' or odd, or strangely negative and resistant, and you wondered what was going on. Sometimes it is only in the post-interview reflection and recording that you can begin to work out what was happening, and how you can best handle it in future.

Exercise 2

Think about someone with whom you have developed a professional relationship. Were there occasions within that relationship where you wondered 'What was going on'? Do you feel that transference was taking place in some ways? How did you handle it? How might you have handled it better?

This would be a good exercise to undertake with an experienced colleague, supervisor or practice teacher.

Other aspects

There are, however, other aspects to developing a professional relationship beyond the work you do with people who come to you and your agency. Two aspects will demand your attention: your professional relationship with your colleagues within your agency, and also with colleagues in other agencies. Each of these deserves careful attention.

Professional relationships with colleagues in your agency

There are almost as many styles of team-working among professional people-workers as there are people to populate them. If you have had experience of working in several teams, you will know that each of them has had its own unique culture. This will affect how colleagues relate to each other and to their manager(s); how they treat administrative and secretarial colleagues, and the extent to which team-working is a stated objective to be worked at in specific ways, as opposed to a loose description of a group of workers who happen to inhabit a particular building. Individual characteristics quickly emerge in a team, and in larger teams sub-groups sometimes form (referred to as cliques by those who are not part of them); occasionally deep friendships are forged. Jealousies sometimes come to the surface, especially when there is a contested promotion opportunity; powerful personalities can seek to dominate other team members. By contrast, teams can also bring the best out of people by creating a supportive, creative and challenging environment in which individuals not only seek to do their best; they sometimes exceed their own expectations as the team culture strives for and achieves excellence.

Whatever your present team is like, there remains an underlying important principle to be observed: that you, and everyone else, must be committed to developing and maintaining professional relationships with everyone else in the team. This does not mean that you will necessarily like everyone or agree with them: that would be naive and unrealistic. But it does mean that you will need to:

- Ensure that you know what your role is; why you are there, and what your function is within the team and with those whom your agency seeks to work.
- Avoid inappropriate relationships within the team: you need to treat everyone with dignity and respect.
- Avoid rumour-mongering, back-biting and putting other colleagues down.
- Ensure that your own standard of work is always the best you can achieve.
- Ensure that other people can take over your work quickly and effectively if necessary: good accurate and up-to-date record keeping is essential.
- Consult and seek advice where appropriate, and make effective use of supervision.
- Contribute to the discussions and consultations within the team, making your own contributions clearly but respecting what others say, and ensuring that you carry out agreed decisions even if you do not wholeheartedly agree with them. It is not your job to undermine the team by niggardly negativism.
- Respect the agreed dress code and other cultural aspects of the team's behaviour. If you need to challenge aspects of this, do it in an

open way through team meetings or raising it with your manager in an open, honest way.

- Develop strategies for leaving your work worries 'at work', and not letting them distort your personal and private life.

- Give due regard to your own personal safety especially when seeing people in their own homes or in unsupervised settings. If you work beyond the end of office hours and have not returned to work, make sure that you use the reporting system to inform your 'buddy' or designated colleague that you are safe and are going home. Make sure before you leave that the office staff know where you are going and what you are planning to do. This is for your own safety.

- Ensure that you plan and take your annual leave entitlement. This is to ensure that you do not risk experiencing 'burn out', and that as far as can reasonably be expected, you are fresh and at your best to do your job effectively at all times.

- Notify your manager if there are issues of a personal nature that prevent your doing your job properly. The boundary between 'personal' and 'professional' is not always easy to maintain, and if you are feeling particularly stressed or unable to function effectively you owe it to yourself, your manager, your agency and to those who come to you for help to be open and honest about this, and to see how you can best be supported through difficult times.

- Do not give out any information about any of your colleagues to anyone else, however plausible their request may seem. Personal information, including contact details, are to remain personal and confidential. You may offer to pass a message on to your colleague, and ask the colleague to contact the enquirer direct. It may sometimes also be appropriate to give them a colleague's official work-issued mobile telephone number. But personal contact details must never be divulged. To do this would be a sure-fire way of losing the confidence and respect of your colleagues, who would have every right to lodge a complaint against you for unprofessional conduct.

- There have been occasions in some teams where the close working relationships between colleagues have developed into intimate friendships and sexual relationships. There are no absolute rules about this, but there are clear 'best practice' guidelines should this happen. These include (1) notifying your manager about your relationship and being open and honest with them about it; (2) ensuring that the personal and professional boundaries are scrupulously observed in the workplace, so that your relationships with other colleagues and those who use your agency's services are not compromised in any way.

Exercise 3

Spend some time working through the checklist given above and undertake a personal 'audit' about how you fare against each of the points raised. Are there any glaring issues that cause you concern? If so, how will you go about addressing them?

Professional relationships with other agencies

It is important to remember that each time you contact another agency in a professional capacity you are acting as the 'face' and representative of your own agency. How you deal with others will, in some measure at least, confirm or diminish the reputation of your agency in the other person's eyes. Your professionalism (or lack of it) is therefore an important aspect of what you will be communicating to others.

How best to achieve this is not difficult, but it does involve following some basic guidelines. These include:

- Stating clearly who you are and which agency you represent. If meeting people face to face, you need to show your ID card or badge to confirm your identity and 'bona fides' if you are meeting them for the first time.
- Observe all the professional courtesies about arriving to meetings/ appointments on time, and observing the appropriate dress code.
- Ensure that you are well prepared: have key information at your fingertips, and say clearly why you need to be in touch with the other agency.
- Recognise and practise confidentiality. This may involve giving your contact details to the other agency for them to ring you back so that your 'bona fides' can be verified. After all, anyone can ring an agency and give false personal details and seek to gain confidential information. If in doubt, write a formal letter asking for the information you require on official letter head, or via a secure intranet.
- If you are leaving messages, give your name, your agency, the date, time and reason for calling, and remember to leave contact details for them to ring back.
- Always do your best to return messages from other agencies as promptly as you can.
- If you have cause to complain about a colleague in another agency, seek advice and guidance from your manager beforehand so that you can be guided into the most appropriate course of action.

- Do not get embroiled in 'slagging off' colleagues from other agencies (or within your own agency), however justified you may feel their bad practice has been. If there are serious issues of malpractice, consult your manager in the first instance to decide on how most appropriately to act, including a consideration of whistle blowing.
- If you are contacted by the press or media representatives about an issue, explain politely that you are not in a position to make a comment, but that you will ask a senior manager to get back to them if they give you their contact details.
- If you receive telephone calls asking for information about someone whom your agency is working with, remember the golden rule about confidentiality. Ask them to put their request in writing if you are unsure about their 'bona fides'. Always explain that you are not at liberty to divulge information about anyone without clear permission.

Final thoughts

The relationship you establish with someone whom you are seeking to help, support or advise in a professional capacity is crucial to the success of your work. If you get it right, then you stand a good chance of 'being part of the solution'; if you get it wrong, then almost certainly you will have become 'part of the problem'. It is as important as that.

Further reading

Harrison, R. et al. (2003) *Partnership Made Painless: A Joined-Up Guide to Working Together*. Lyme Regis: Russell House Publishing.

Martin, V. and Henderson, E. (2001) *Managing in Health and Social Care*. Abingdon: Routledge.

Thompson, N. (2006) *Promoting Workplace Learning*. Bristol: The Policy Press.

Trevithick, P. (2005) *Social Work Skills – A Practice Handbook*. Maidenhead: Open University Press.

Related concepts   Confidentiality; endings; non-verbal communication; reflective practice; supervision; whistle blowing.

Feedback – Giving and Receiving

Feedback is the verbal or written evaluation of someone's performance; a comment on how well or otherwise they have done in completing a particular task. Feedback therefore requires excellent communication skills to be effective.

People-work provides many opportunities for feedback, as the following list demonstrates:

- a supervisor comments upon a trainee's interview which was formally observed and assessed
- a worker comments on a task that had been given to a user of the services during their previous interview
- a colleague asks you to say what you think of the draft report they have just written;
- your manager evaluates your performance over the past three months.

These are but a few of the occasions where feedback is used, and almost always it carries with it the opportunity to suggest how performance can be enhanced or improved. In other words, it can be a valuable tool in promoting and facilitating best practice.

This assumes, however, that it is both given and received in the right way. Poor feedback can often be a disincentive to improvement, although there are occasions when being told 'you are no good' at something can spur some people on to greater efforts 'just to show them that they are wrong'. Within a professional context, however, such a tactic is rarely, if ever, justifiable.

Oral feedback

One important starting point for this discussion is the tendency with many people, when asked how they got on with, let us say, conducting a particular interview, to say that 'it was dreadful' or, 'I was hopeless'. The aspects of the interview which they feel did not go well, rise to the surface first. But such negativity rarely serves to improve practice; it may even be the rather immature behaviour of a child seeking a parent's approval, comfort and reassurance, rather than an adult-to-adult, genuine quest for improvement.

The general guidelines for giving feedback, therefore, encourage you to take a different approach, both for giving feedback to someone else, and also when evaluating your own performance. These guidelines are sometimes known as 'Pendleton's rules', and are carefully followed particularly in medical circles when giving feedback to trainee doctors who are developing their communication skills. They are, however, relevant to all feedback in people-work.

The key point to make with Pendleton's (1984) approach is that we all tend to learn more, better and faster, if we have the positive aspects of our performance identified and confirmed first of all. Therefore, a typical first question to ask will be, 'What went well in that interview?' or, 'Tell me what pleased you most about how you conducted that interview.' This approach immediately invites you to think about positives, even if that feels a very difficult thing to do. There will always be things that went well, which will be strengths to build on. When these have been identified, then you can move on to ask, not what was bad about it, but rather, 'How might you have done it differently?' or, 'If you had the chance to do this again, how do you think you might improve on what you have just done?' This again puts the focus on best practice, and encourages you to think creatively about the skills you have used. Again, there will almost always be things which could have been done differently: after all, there is no such thing as a perfect interview!

Not that these guidelines are to be followed absolutely slavishly. If, for example, someone has made a real hash of an interview, it would be foolish to spend so much time on the few positive aspects of it that there was not enough time really to focus on how the interview should be improved. People-workers spend their professional lives working with vulnerable people, and it is imperative that in the training scenario maximum use is made of the opportunity to fine-tune these skills and approaches. Better that someone's pride is a bit dented in the safe environment of a training event than making serious mistakes for real that could have been avoided had the trainer identified problem areas, and suggested ways of doing things better.

As part of this aspect of the feedback, therefore, it is sometimes helpful to identify any points in the interview where the interviewer felt they were floundering, or got stuck, or panicked. These moments can be replayed in the discussion, and suggestions made for how such situations could be handled differently. These are the ways in which we can develop our communication skills and develop best practice.

Feedback on written work

The same approach applies also to giving feedback on written work. It is always helpful to give an overall impression about the piece of work by saying what you particularly liked about the way it was written, or its style, or its clarity of thought. You can then move on to suggest how other aspects of it could be developed, or the style modified. Sometimes, for example, people forget the audience for which the report is being prepared. Formal reports call for formal language, whereas some letters need to adopt a far more casual, informal tone to get the right meaning across.

Mis-spellings and poor grammar always need to be addressed. Usually a light-hearted suggestion that they run this through the computer's spell-check or grammar check before sending it out will do the trick. But sometimes, where issues of dyslexia are involved, you may want to check carefully that the person has had a proper assessment and has access to one of the many computerised packages which are designed to enable people for whom dyslexia is an issue, to produce good, accurate pieces of written work.

There is, however, one important caveat to all of this. There is a corrective function to feedback that clearly must come into play if the interviewer has given incorrect information during the course of the interview. This is clearly an important role for the tutor to play in giving feedback, so that incorrect or inaccurate information is not left unchallenged.

Some more principles

These comments highlight another important principle in giving feedback. The comments should always focus on the behaviour (e.g., the conduct of an interview) or the end product (e.g., a written piece of work), but *not* the person. Feedback is not another term for character assassination: it is based on the assumption that the person will have done their best, albeit often in difficult circumstances, and what each of you wants from feedback is an acknowledgement of what went well and how performance could be improved.

Another important principle is that feedback should be given as soon as possible after it has been requested. If it is feedback on an interview, for example, the person giving feedback should try to give some immediate response as soon after the event as possible, using the principles outlined above. This could be quite brief, but it puts the person out of their suspense. More detailed feedback can follow at an agreed day and time. If it is feedback on a written piece of work, there should be some discussion about when the feedback can be given and how. Would the person prefer this to be done verbally, or would comments written on the document be perfectly adequate?

Role play feedback

In training people for professional people-work, the use of role play, especially with simulated patients/service users, is becoming increasingly popular in medical and social work education, for example. The reason for this is clear: there are limitations to the extent to which students in training can accurately play the role of someone in need. It will feel far more authentic if an 'outsider' to the group comes in to role play the scenarios. Feedback in such training sessions can be much more detailed, not least because the trainer/observer, the trainee and the role player can all be invited to give feedback. This is what makes these exercises valuable, because everyone's perspective can be explored.

Pendleton suggests the following 'rules' or guidelines for such scenarios:

1 When the interview has finished, the interviewer is asked to comment on what went well, and this is followed by the role player giving their feedback, still in role. For example, 'As the service user in this interview I felt that you really made me feel at ease by the way you looked attentively at me, and asked me if I felt comfortable.'
2 Following this, the observer/trainer gives feedback, with specific examples of what went well.
3 The interviewer next has an opportunity to suggest what might have been done differently, and how certain aspects of the interview might have been handled in a different way.
4 This then provides the role player, still in role, to comment on this, and make their own suggestions of what might have been helpful at various points in the interview, and how this might have felt.
5 The observer/trainer then can add comments about how things might have been handled differently.
6 Finally, with the role player coming out of role, there can be a rounding-off discussion to clarify the learning points that have been identified. These points need to be specific and detailed so that the interviewer can use the feedback to improve on specific aspects of their performance.

These guidelines maximise the opportunity for constructive feedback, and can play a crucial role in helping trainees develop their communication skills.

Exercise 1

If you are a trainee, the chances are that you will be directly observed during your training. Next time you have feedback from your trainer, check that these guidelines are being followed. Check also how the feedback makes you feel, and to what extent it is going to help you improve your practice. Then give this feedback to your trainer, using the guidelines we have provided.

Exercise 2

If you are a more experienced worker, find an opportunity when you are giving feedback, and double-check to see that you are following these guidelines. Then after you have given the feedback, ask for feedback on how you gave the feedback! if you do not ask, you will not find out!

Final thoughts

This discussion is a reminder that you never work in a vacuum, and that communication skills are always a shared, corporate activity. We constantly need to check out whether what we are trying to communicate and achieve is actually working. Therefore, the feedback mirror is always an essential part of your toolbox, so that you can assess with the help of others how effective you are in the work you are undertaking.

References and Further reading

Pendelton, D. et al. (1984) *The Consultation: An Approach to Learning*. Oxford: Oxford University Press. (see chapter 5, Analysing interviews and giving feedback in experiential teaching sessions)

Thompson, N. (2006) *Promoting Workplace Learning*. Bristol: The Policy Press.

Trevithick, P. (2005) *Social Work Skills: A Practice Handbook*. 2nd edition Maidenhead: Open University Press. (pp. 169–70 and *passim*)

Related concepts   Active listening; establishing a professional relationship; reflective practice; supervision.

Genograms

The old saying that 'a picture is worth a thousand words' certainly applies to genograms, which are pictorial representations of a set of family relationships. With just a few basic symbols and a set of ground rules, you can quickly capture a lot of important information about the person or family you are working with.

Although genograms are usually associated with therapeutic family work, they can be useful for anyone working with people. They can be used both during or after an interview for the following purposes:

- to summarise the core information which has been gained
- as a working tool to help gain information
- to help understand and interpret information
- to use in case notes to which other workers can refer.

It is important to stress at the outset that anyone using a genogram during an interview must be very familiar with how it works, so that it really is a tool to be used and not a straightjacket which constrains. If it is not helpful to you, then don't use it.

Building block 1

The symbols used in genograms are simple and straightforward.

Relationships are portrayed by lines that link the two (see page 116). So a continuous line represents a stable, even permanent relationship, and a dotted line, a recently established relationship that has not developed into any degree of permanency. If a relationship has ended, the a single slash indicates a separation; a double slash, a divorce.

At this point, some limitations will immediately become clear. There is no obvious distinction between a couple who are legally married and those who have been living together for a period of years. If it is important to know this, then you will need to add written information somewhere on or near the line (e.g., m 27/10/85 could be added for the date of marriage; cp 19/3/07 for the date when a civil partnership was legally recognised).

Already, two important points have emerged. First, pictures only tell us so much; we will need to add brief written notes to clarify or

Building block 1

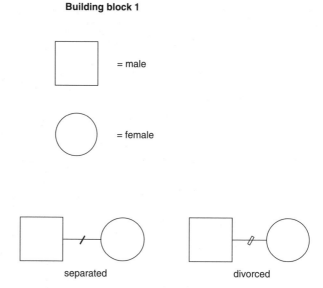

supplement information; and, second, genograms can be used just as effectively for single sex and with heterosexual relationships.

Building block 2: – The family tree

Using the basic building blocks, a family tree can be depicted, with both children and grandparents being located. Additional information can be added to show the ages of the people concerned, and whether or not they are still alive. For example, the genogram below tells us several key facts.

Building block 2

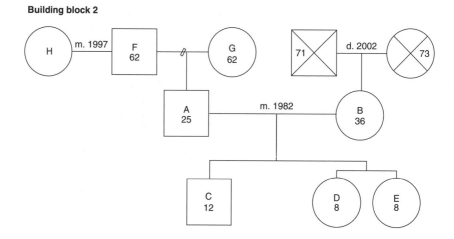

A is 25 years old and is married to B who is 36. They were married in 1982. They have 3 children, C who is a boy aged 12, and twin girls D + E who are 8.

A's parents F + G, both aged 62, are divorced; F married H in 1997, while G still lives alone.

B's parents are both dead; they died in 2002 aged 71 and 73 respectively.

Exercise 1

At this point if you are not familiar with genograms, it is a good idea to 'have a go' for yourself. Do one for your own situation. Start with yourself, and build it up in whatever way you wish, incorporating any siblings you may have; your parents and perhaps grandparents; your partner if you are in a relationship, and children if you have any. You will probably want to have a large sheet of paper to work on.

After you have completed your genogram, you will want to see first of all whether you have used the building blocks and ground rules accurately. This is important because another worker may subsequently need to look at it, and you will want to ensure that you are both speaking the same language with the pictures and symbols you are using.

The next thing likely to emerge is that it was probably not as easy as you thought! You may have wondered how to fit all the information in; or you may have run out of space at the edge of the page and have had to start again. Don't worry! This is a learning curve, and there is no rule to say you have to get it right the first time. But do get some practice in so that you are familiar with how genograms work, and you will soon get the hang of it.

Exercise 2

If you are currently working with someone and have a set of notes and information about them, spend some time trying to express that information in the form of a genogram, when you have some time to spare. Decide what written information you need to add, either on the genogram itself, or in some footnotes in the margin.

(Continued)

(Continued)

When you have finished, show it to an appropriate colleague to see how effectively you have completed it, and whether their interpretation of your genogram matches the facts as you know them.

One further thing to look for – sometimes it is only when we start drawing a picture that we notice the gaps and the things which appear to be missing – it is like an incomplete jigsaw, and it helps us to begin to ask questions about the information we have represented in our diagram. Who are, or might be, the people lurking in the background who have still to be mentioned?

You could, if this is an ongoing piece of work, take your genogram to the next interview or meeting, and explain that you have been trying to get a full picture of the situation. Explain how the genogram system works, then ask them if this is an accurate portrayal; ask then about the gaps which you think are there.

As soon as you start using a genogram *with* someone you are working with, tread very carefully. The information you portray in what may appear to you to be a very straightforward way in simple picture language, may have a powerful impact upon the person whose life is being 'examined'. The gaps may trigger off some emotional reaction when you start to explore them. So always remember that this is a tool that potentially can be very powerful.

The same point needs to be made if genograms are being introduced in a training context. You may find that the very process of seeking out information to complete the genogram can raise painful issues for some people.

Building block 3: Interpreting – making sense – adding meaning

The exercises suggested above, and the accompanying commentary, have taken us into the next level in the use of genograms, that is, the interpretation of the information. This can happen in a variety of ways.

First, we may find that people want to talk about some of the characters who appear in the genogram with a degree of strong feelings. They may love them or loathe them, for example; they may feel very close to them, or very distant from them; there may be some very stressful relationships uncovered.

It is sometimes helpful, therefore, to capture these feelings and the quality of these relationships with some different symbols. For example, the use of a jagged zig-zaggy line between two people would indicate a very stressful relationship, whereas a thick, strong unbroken line between two people would indicate a strong – even affectionate – bond. And if you decided to use different colours on the genogram to emphasise these differing types of relationships, then a powerful picture quickly begins to emerge.

Second, some sensitive questioning about how various people in the overall picture relate to one another may again uncover some shades of meaning about the quality of the relationships and 'who means what to whom' in the overall family tree. By using the same symbols as before, an emotional, much more dynamic picture of the 'family' begins to emerge. Of particular significance may be the barriers between various people that block relationships. You may want to portray the barriers with a strong symbol on the genogram. If such barriers are problematic and trouble the person you are working with (and remember that the barriers may *not* be a problem, so it is not our job to make problems if they do not exist), then this may prompt a discussion about the barriers and how they feel about them and how they might be overcome.

Third, we can place a dotted line around all those who currently live together in the same household.

Final thoughts

It is implicit throughout all the discussion about genograms that you need to be clear in your mind about why you want to use them, and how they can be useful tools in your work with people. If you use them just for your own benefit as an enrichment of your case recording, and as a means of reflecting on issues which have been, or still need to be raised, then you remain very much in charge of the process. Once you start using them in direct work with people, however, it becomes a much more interactive, dynamic, two-way process: that is its strength, but as a worker you need to be fully prepared for it to be a powerful tool in your professional relationships.

As with all tools, genograms have their strengths and their limitations. You may find that it will be helpful to look at the possibility of using ecomaps, for example when you are trying to explore more complex inter-relationships between people.

The golden practice rule in all of this, however, is confidence. If you can introduce genograms into direct work with people in a sensitive, confident way, aware of the potential benefits as well as possible pitfalls, then you are likely to find the use of genograms can considerably enhance your practice.

Further reading

Coulshed, V. and Orme, J. (2006) *Social Work Practice*. 4th
  edition. Basingstoke: Palgrave Macmillan.
Compton, B. and Galaway, B. (1989) *Social Work Processes*. 4th
  edition. Belmont, California: Wadsworth Publishing Co.
www.smartdraw.com
www.multiculturalfamily.org/genograms

Related concepts   Ecomaps; partnership working; reflective practice.

Getting Unstuck

There is hardly a people-worker in existence who has not had the
unnerving experience while interviewing someone of feeling completely and utterly 'stuck'. The interviewee has dried up and become
silent, you have lost track of where the interview is going, you can't
think of what to say next, and you wish that the ground would open
up and swallow you up. It is a very unnerving and uncomfortable
experience.

Although there are no foolproof solutions, it is often possible to free
the logjam by using some tried and tested techniques before having
recourse to the ultimate strategy of 'calling it a day' and deciding that
no further progress can be made on this occasion.

Much will depend, of course, on the context of the interview. For
example, an uncommunicative young person may feel overwhelmed by
having to come to an austere office to meet someone old enough to be
a parent or grandparent. In such circumstances, if no progress is being
made, a change of venue or a younger worker may free up the communications. If, however, a person comes for an appointment under the
influence of alcohol or other substances, it is probably wise not even to
begin to interview them, but rather to give them another appointment
and ask them to come in sober and clear-headed next time. There are
also occasions when progress in an interview is minimal because the

person you are seeking to interview is accompanied by someone who 'puts a damper' on the occasion. A young person accompanied by a parent or relative may not wish to disclose information or feelings in front of that person and will retreat into a sullen silence to make precisely that point. In such circumstances, if alternative accommodation is available, and the setting is safe, the worker may suggest that just the two of them have some time together without the parental figure being in the same room. You may also find that on some home visits there are other people or children present, in front of whom the person you wish to interview quite appropriately feels unable to open up and discuss things with you.

These are some examples where the experience of getting stuck – or sometimes not even getting started – are due to circumstantial and contextual factors which need to be acknowledged and dealt with. Change the circumstances and you may well find that conversation begins to flow freely. Inevitably this may mean abandoning the first meeting in favour of a second one in a more conducive setting, and this may annoy or frustrate you. But it is far better to recognise the barriers to communication at that point rather than try to soldier on and find yourself becoming increasingly alienated from the other person.

There are also some other 'barrier moments' that are more challenging, and will call for sensitive handling. For example:

- you are a white male worker and find yourself being asked to work with a married Asian woman
- you are a black worker and find yourself in the presence of a white service user who 'point blank' refuses to be seen by someone who is black
- you are trying to work with someone for whom English is not their first language, and who clearly struggles to communicate with you
- a learning-disabled person with verbal communication difficulties becomes increasingly angry and frustrated at not being able to let you know what they need.

Exercise 1

Spend a few moments considering each of the scenarios outlined above. What do you feel is the best-practice response? Where do you think the barriers to communication lie in each of these scenarios? What can be done to get 'unstuck'?

In these scenarios, it can be argued that in three of them the reasons for becoming stuck lie in the structural inequality of the relationship and the barriers that in some ways, wittingly or unwittingly, the worker erects. In such situations, best practice would suggest that an early attempt to remove such barriers will be a necessary pre-condition to meaningful communication. Ideally, a female Asian worker might be able to make significantly more progress than the original white male worker about whom the woman is likely to feel a strong measure of cultural diffidence and a reluctance to confide. Similarly, to provide effective communication assistance, by way of an interpreter, or an appropriate communication board, may provide the breakthrough to better communication in two of the other scenarios.

More problematic is the situation where someone refuses a service on grounds of 'race'. Here the barrier is clearly located in the prejudice and racist attitudes of the person coming to the agency. The main question here is whether the agency should be seen to collude with these attitudes and provide a white worker instead, or whether the issue is so fundamental to the value-base of the agency that they will say to the person that not only are such attitudes unacceptable to them, but also that the person must choose whether to accept the service from this worker or not to have any service at all. This is clearly an issue where the agency must have a very clear policy so that individual workers are fully supported in the decisions that are taken in such situations.

These are some of the contextual barriers that may cause you to feel 'stuck' when trying to conduct an interview. It goes without saying that until these barriers are removed to a greater or lesser extent, no meaningful communication will be possible.

Within an interview that has begun to make some progress, however, the possibility of getting 'stuck' is all too real. There are no automatic guaranteed 'unblocking' techniques, although some of the following 'tried and tested' approaches often yield some success. These are offered in no particular order of importance. The first two, summarising and paraphrasing, are basic skills you will want to use generally in your active listening skills, as they are useful techniques to facilitate progress during an interview, whether or not there are moments of getting stuck.

Summarising   It is useful when stuck to use the basic skill of summarising the story so far. You must find the forms of words which suits you best, but something like this is what we have in mind: 'J, I wonder if it will help if I try to put into my words what you have been telling me?' and then after you have had an attempt at doing this, ask something like 'Have I got it right, J?' or 'Is that how it feels?' or 'Is this what you are trying to say to me?'

The chances are that this will take some of the pressure off, and allow the other person to listen to you. In some ways it does not matter if you do not get it 100 per cent right: they will quickly tell you if you have misinterpreted or misrepresented them, and that can give a fresh impetus to the interview.

Paraphrasing   This is a similar skill to summarising, except that with paraphrasing you do not need to try to deal with the whole story so far. Instead you can take perhaps just the last point the other person was trying to make, and reflect it back to them in your own words. For example, 'J, have I got this right? You seem to be saying to me that you hate your father's guts?'

Again, this mirroring back provides an opportunity for the other person to discover how well you have been listening to them and how they have come across to you.

Acknowledging being stuck   This may seem an obvious point to make, but sometimes it is the simplest things that work best. A range of statements or questions can be used to nudge the logjam, such as:

J, have you run out of things to say?

J, you seem really stuck – are you finding it difficult to continue?

J, I wish I could help you carry on talking to me.

What is it, J? You seem lost for words.

Are you struggling with something really difficult to tell me, J?

J, would you like a short break before we carry on?

J, would you prefer to carry on with this on another occasion?

J, I think you have done really well in getting this far – it doesn't surprise me that you want a bit of a breather.

J, is there anything else you want to say today?

Sharing the silence   Sometimes we fall into the trap of thinking that every moment must be filled with words; we find it hard to acknowledge that we find silences difficult to cope with, and that it is our needs which are being met when we want to kickstart the conversation as quickly as possible. It is just possible, however, that the other person's lapse into silence is no more, but certainly no less, than a pause for reflection. In such situations, you will probably help most if you stay quiet and allow the other person to have some space. Initially, no words are necessary, so long as you maintain a caring, interested body posture to help them appreciate that you are still 'with them' and are concerned for them. Judging when a silence probably needs to be broken, albeit gently, is a real skill, but you will gain some clues by the body language and general attitude of the other person. If they are clearly looking thoughtful and reflective and perhaps upset, it may be helpful to allow the silence to continue. You may also wish to encourage them by such comments as:

It's OK to take some time out, you know.

Take your time – there's no rush.

You've told me a lot today – perhaps it's important to be quiet for a while to see where we go next.

You don't have to talk you know – it's OK to be quiet for a bit.

I'm glad you feel able to be silent with me – not everyone can do that.

If, on the other hand, they are themselves restless, and are gazing round the room and looking bored, that tells you that you need to re-engage quickly, and some of the summarising or paraphrasing techniques may help. But you may also want to face them with their apparent boredom in a direct way. For example:

J, you are beginning to look a bit bored – have you had enough?

J, can you help me – I'm not sure where we go from here?

Are you wishing you were somewhere else, J?

I suppose your teacher at school would've told you off if you'd looked as bored in class as you do now!

Come on, J – you're doing OK – let's have another go!

Half time's over, J – time to come out for the second half!

Are you still here, J?

Final thoughts

The very nature of people-work means that no one can tell you exactly how to deal with difficult moments like getting stuck; and perversely, no matter much you seek to prepare yourself, when the moment comes, the feeling of being stuck is so real and genuine that it is not easy to break out of it. Nevertheless, it is useful to have some of these techniques up your sleeve so that you can 'oil the wheels' of the interview and help it come to a satisfactory conclusion. But if all else fails and you do not effect a breakthrough, there is no harm in suggesting that you call a halt for today and arrange a further appointment. In such circumstances it is helpful to acknowledge that you realise that they, and you, have found the interview difficult, and that next time you would like them to come prepared to talk about whatever topics or themes that seem to be important. You might also like to pose a question for them to take away to help them prepare for next time. You can also offer to reflect on what might be most useful to think about next time, so that there is a sense of a shared responsibility for making next time become more productive for you both.

Further reading

Kadushin, A. (1997) *The Social Work Interview – A Guide for Human Service Professionals*. 4th edition. New York: Columbia University Press.

Thompson, N. (2002) *People Skills*. 2nd edition Basingtoke: Palgrave Macmillan.

Trevithick, P. (2005) *Social Work Skills – A Practice Handbook*. 2nd edition. Maidenhead: Open University Press.

Related concepts   Active listening skills; barrier gestures; endings; non-verbal communication; interpreters; reflective practice.

Information Technology (IT)

There has been an explosion of information made available in recent years, principally through the Internet. With the click of a mouse we can discover information about almost anything. Whether this information is accurate is another matter, but it is beyond doubt that the 'mouse' rules supreme. Even that statement is somewhat dated, as new mobile technologies come on stream and you can access whatever you want from the palm of your hand.

IT developments have transformed the ways in which people-workers operate. Records are now kept electronically. Some organisations equip their workers with laptops so that records may be accessed and updated instantly, and key information gathered and shared during the course of an interview. Social workers now have to be computer literate and to have reached the standard of the European Computer Driving Licence (ECDL) before they can graduate. The facilities provided by email can now enable fast, multiple communications to be exchanged. Within the National Health Service huge changes are being introduced to facilitate the electronic storage of patients' records, choice of hospitals for treatment, and electronic prescriptions

IT developments have facilitated information exchange and have taken communication skills into a new era for professional people-workers. There are some general rules and guidelines which need to be carefully observed, however, if this new era is not to be counter-productive. These include:

- Professional people-workers need to keep to the quality standards and protocols laid down by their agency for everything to do with IT.
- Agency IT facilities exist for the benefit of the agency and the people it serves: they are not there for individual and personal use by the employees.
- Inappropriate use of emails (e.g., to harass others or to send offensive messages or materials) or the Internet (e.g., to surf for pornographic material or even to book your holidays) is unacceptable and liable to lead to disciplinary procedures.

- When sending emails, observe the proper protocols of stating the subject of the email and ensure that your details are correctly cited in your personal signature section. Be concise, but not terse: remember the courtesies, and do not forget to thank people for their responses. You will find that various agencies have their own house-style for emails.
- Special care must be taken to ensure confidentiality is maintained in all electronic communications; you should not leave sensitive information displayed on your screen if you leave your desk unattended. You should not be transferring any official information from agency machines to your personal machines at home. If you need to do work at home that involves electronic technology, you should seek the guidance and written permission from your manager.
- You should not bring material on floppy disks or 'memory sticks' into your agency and transfer it to the office equipment without specific permission, and then only after virus checks have been scrupulously undertaken. One virus could wipe out masses of information, and if this is your fault, you will face disciplinary procedures.
- Be sure that you understand how your own agency IT system works, and be sure to follow procedures carefully, especially with regards to saving and storing information.
- You should be encouraged to use the Internet to access relevant sources of information. For example, key Government and research agency websites will enable you to keep up-to-date with recent developments and policy changes that you will need for your practice. More general access to a wider range of websites will need to be undertaken with a degree of circumspection, however, so that you are sure of their 'bona fides' and the reliability of their information.

Exercise 1

This is an opportunity for you to conduct a personal audit of your IT skills and how you use them as part of your professional practice.

- List the ways in which you and your agency use IT.
- What areas do you feel confident and competent in using?
- What areas of personal development in IT do you feel would help you do your job better? How could you access training to achieve this improvement?

Final thoughts

Computers and IT can enrich our professional service delivery, but they should not replace the essential human contact between people, which is the life blood of any organisation that works with people.

Further reading

Gregor, C. (2006) *Practical Computer Skills for Social Work.* Exeter: Learning Matters.
Moran, J., Hull, V. and Wheeler, D. (2003) *The Complete Idiot's Guide to ECDL.* London: Prentice Hall.
Munnelly, B. and Holden, P. (2005) *ECDL 4: The Complete Course Book for Microsoft 2003.* Harlow, Pearson Education Ltd: Prentice Hall.

Interpreters

In a multicultural society there is an increasingly important emphasis to be placed upon the availability of interpreters so that people for whom English is not their first language may have their needs and requirements accurately addressed.

Interpreting, of course, is a much wider communication than this initial definition suggests. In any communication between and among people, there will be a continual process of interpreting as we try to make sense of what the other person is seeking to communicate. How we interpret non-verbal communication or barrier gestures are good examples of this: we need to check whether the meaning we are giving to their message is accurate or not; or to put it another way, whether we are accurately interpreting what the other person is saying or doing. Interpreting therefore is a fundamental, generalist skill that underlies and underpins all communication.

This skill comes into sharper focus, however, when issues around language are involved. Not only are there the general challenges about understanding what the other person is saying: there is also the added challenge of translating this message from one language to another in order for it to be properly received.

Exercise 1

Think about the work you do and the demographic make-up of the area your agency covers. Do you know how many different cultural groups there are, and therefore how many different languages are in general use in the area? Do you know how many people are not able to converse with agencies using English? How many would much prefer to have the use of a skilled interpreter so that they can explain what they need in their first language? If you find these questions difficult to answer, how might you go about finding out more information?

Your responses to the above exercise will have been informative, and will have given you some idea of the size and scope of the challenge your agency faces. There is considerable political debate, of course, about the extent to which everyone in the UK should have a sufficiently clear grasp of English in order to access services effectively. But the issue is more complex than that. In Wales, for example, it has been a matter of pride and national/cultural identity that people should be given the choice as to whether they access information and services in Welsh or English. It is a similar principle and value-base that is behind the drive to extend this choice to other cultural groups within society.

There are additional issues to consider. Deaf people, for example, for whom British Sign Language (BSL) is their first language, do not have the option of linguistic choice. BSL is their language, and there is a responsibility and legal obligation upon organisations to ensure that Deaf people can access information and services.

British Sign Language is a good example to explore, because it highlights some of the key issues of interpretation and indeed translation that underlie all attempts to convey meaning accurately from one language to another. With BSL there is a structural issue to take into account, because it is such a visual means of communication. The most obvious example that is familiar to anyone learning basic BSL is how you ask someone else's name. 'What's your name?' seems an easy enough question to pose, but in BSL the literal translation would be, 'Your name, what?', because the visual message needs to have a different structure in order to make it more quickly comprehensible. A system of 'multi-channel' signs in BSL ensures that a broad range of complex communication can be shared quickly and easily without having recourse to a laborious finger-spelling of every single word.

For someone to be an effective interpreter for a Deaf person, therefore, they not only need a deep knowledge of two languages, but also an ability to move between them quickly and fluently so that the real meaning behind the words or symbols can be effectively communicated.

This example illustrates the complexity of an interpreter's task. In some languages and cultures there may not be an equivalent or comparable word for such terms as depression, dementia or counselling, for example, and the interpreter may have a difficult task in trying to convey and translate what is meant. Indeed, there may have to be a discussion between the worker and the interpreter so that the worker is 'brought up to speed' with the problems that certain words, terms and phrases are causing.

This highlights two key principles behind all interpreting: trust and accuracy.

Trust

The issue of trust is paramount, and is two-sided. For example, a woman whose first language is Punjabi may be accompanied by her husband or another male family member who will act as interpreter for the interview. There is no doubt that if that family member has a command of English, good interpretation is possible. But a female worker may feel that issues of gender and culture may become a barrier to accurate communication. She may not be sure whether the male family member is at times speaking on behalf of the woman, as opposed to being the mouthpiece for the woman. She may begin to wonder whether she can really trust the process of interpretation.

For this reason, it is considered best practice in all people-work for an official, accredited interpreter to be made available for such interviews, and indeed for other official and formal occasions such as court appearances or meetings with local authority officials. The interpreter's code of conduct should ensure that good accurate communication takes place, especially as factors such as gender and 'race' are taken into account in the choice of interpreter to be employed for this purpose.

There can, of course, be no absolute guarantee of this, not least because communication is such a complex phenomenon. But every agency should have access to an interpreter scheme to ensure that these basic issues can be properly and effectively addressed, and that both 'parties' feel that they can trust the interpreter to do the job honestly and accurately and without any personal prejudice.

Accuracy

The principle of accuracy is also fundamental, and underlies the capacity of each person to understand the other. From the worker's point of view it is important to establish some appropriate guidelines and ground-rules before an interview or meeting begins. These include:

- Checking that the other person is happy with the interpreter and can trust them to communicate their views and opinions honestly and accurately;
- Checking that the interpreter knows the ground-rules and code of conduct, and is willing to translate and interpret accurately even if the views and opinions which are being interpreted go against their own personal or cultural convictions;
- Agreeing the boundaries and whether it is acceptable for the interpreter to begin to plead the cause of the other person in addition to the role of interpeter, and to be clear when this is being undertaken;
- Explaining the structure of the interaction, by giving an undertaking that the interview will not be hurried; that the conversation will be conducted in 'bite-size chunks' that are easily manageable, and that on a regular basis the worker will pause to check that everything is clear;
- Encouraging the other person to say at any point if they do not understand what is being said or asked of them;
- Encouraging written notes to be made in each language about key points being made; it is good practice for each person to have a copy of the notes in each language for future reference.

Working with interpreters is an important skill that needs practice. It is useful to discuss this with colleagues who have already developed these skills, and if possible to seek permission to sit in on and observe another interview where an interpreter is being used so that you can 'get the feel' of what is involved before you have to do it 'for real' yourself.

User perspectives

A criticism of the discussion so far could be that it seems to be from an agency or service-provider perspective; it might even be argued somewhat cynically that these procedures are there to 'cover the backs' of the professional workers in case things go wrong. Such a response would be unwarranted and unfair: best practice is best practice, and there are good reasons underpinning the approaches that have so far been outlined. Nevertheless, any approach that does not fully take into account the user's perspective is bound to feel somewhat 'one-sided', and a negation of the basic principle of partnership-working at the heart of all people-work.

Some important research was conducted by Alexander et al. (2004) with multicultural communities in London and Manchester. Their findings highlighted some important issues for all people-work by drawing attention to the following responses from people who needed interpreters:

- The decision about whether or not an interpreter was necessary should be decided by the people themselves, depending on the situation they were facing. Often they felt they could manage perfectly well by themselves or with their own chosen interpreter, but in legal and medical matters the importance of a trained interpreter was emphasised.
- People expected their interpreters to have good people skills, and where necessary to be able and willing to 'go the extra mile' and plead their cause for them. The personal qualities of trustworthiness and reliability were seen to be crucial. Where these qualities were clearly evident, high expectations were placed on the interpreter to be an effective advocate as well as interpreter, to achieve results from a service provider which seemed better at witholding services than granting them.
- There was considerable difficulty in accessing good quality interpreters in these areas, so that many people preferred family and friends to undertake this role because they felt they could rely on their loyalty and emotional commitment.

These findings demonstrate how important it is for there to be an open and honest dialogue right at the outset to explore the issues of trust and accuracy, what is going to work best for the other person, and also what is best going to serve the legitimate needs of the agency. To explore these issues effectively will require good communication and listening skills, but if handled sensitively will ensure that a good outcome can be achieved.

Final thoughts

Perhaps the only way in which you will fully understand the importance of interpreters is to be in a situation where you need one yourself – perhaps on holiday in a country where you do not speak their language, and have some sort of crisis. You then will need to have someone who is able to help you to become fully involved in the negotiations so that you know exactly what is happening and what is involved. That perhaps will give you an insight into how important at the emotional as well as practical level good quality interpreting is.

References and Further reading

Alexander, C. et al. (2004) *Access to Services with Interpreters: User Views*. York: Joseph Rowntree Foundation.
www.aafp.org. *Family Practice Management. Getting the Most from Language Interpreters*. American Academy of Family Physicians
www.just communication.co.uk

Related concepts   Anti-discriminatory practice; establishing a professional relationship; partnership working.

Interviewing

This whole book, in some way, deals with the basic skills of interviewing. From the moment you welcome someone for the first time, to how you bring the meeting to a close; from how you ask questions and gather information, to how your non-verbal communication makes an impact; all of these communication skills are at the heart of interviewing.

Perhaps as you read the various entries in the book you will be asking whether it applies equally to adults and to children. After all, people-work spans all ages. In many ways the answer to this question is 'yes': many of the skills, and certainly the value-base, apply equally to everyone you interview, no matter what their age is. There are nevertheless some specific issues involved with interviewing children which deserve special attention.

Interviewing children

However complex the interviewing process may be with adults, when children are involved there are additional layers of complexity that must be taken into account, no matter what area of professional practice the worker represents. Social workers, family mediators, doctors, health visitors, nurses, police officers and probation officers: these and many other professionals will, from time to time, be required formally to interview children, and it is of crucial importance that the careful guidelines for good practice are scrupulously followed. This is particularly important where there are cases of child abuse to be investigated. The Memorandum of Good Practice (1992) was introduced by the Home Office as a direct result of the Cleveland Inquiry (1987) and the concerns that were raised following investigations by social workers in Rochdale and Orkney following widespread allegations of sexual abuse.

The worrying background to this discussion, with the many examples of social workers, police officers and paediatric consultants not always achieving best practice, and not always communicating effectively together, has led to a difficult climate in which to work with children. Professional workers find themselves constantly looking over their shoulders, hoping they 'don't get it wrong – again', and many professionals in the field of children's work report high levels of stress and anxiety as they seek to fulfil their obligations and responsibilities.

The difficult climate for this work should not blind you, however, to its crucial importance. One of the hallmarks of a civilised, caring society is the way in which vulnerable people are regarded and respected, and the ways in which children and young people are cherished, valued and encouraged to live their lives to their fullest potential. Anyone who exploits or abuses children is not only damaging the individual child: they are also undermining the basic societal values which cherish children and their place in society. The duty – some would also say privilege – of protecting children is therefore of paramount importance, and just because there are inherent difficulties in the task does not mean we should ever flinch from it.

Exercise 1

Think about some of the work with children you have done, or might be called upon to undertake in your professional capacity. In what ways do you think children can be at risk? Make a list of situations and factors that can put children at risk.

Exercise 2

Think about your role as a worker with children. What are the good and positive aspects of this work? What are the negative aspects of it, or the 'down side' of the work? When you have completed this list, use it as a basis for discussion with your supervisor or practice

(Continued)

(Continued)

teacher. This will help you gain a better picture not only of the work itself, but also of how you are approaching it, what your strengths are, and the aspects of the work that make you feel nervous or inadequate.

When we think about work with children, it is important not to begin with the children, but with ourselves as workers. This involves not only an awareness of the skills we will need to do the work, but also a heightened awareness of ourselves and how we come across to others. It is, admittedly, extremely difficult to see ourselves 'through a child's or young person's eyes', but some attempt must be made as part of our commitment to anti-discriminatory practice and to being reflective practitioners. In the section on non-verbal communication mention is made of how we can communicate a wide range of messages to other people, and this is particularly true when we work with young people. If a child has had their trust in adults undermined or destroyed, it is hardly surprising that they may regard you with some suspicion simply because you are an adult, however different you may be from the adult who has betrayed their trust. You will be seen as a powerful adult, and you will need to practise the communication skills of establishing trust before any meaningful work can be undertaken.

If you are honest, your work with children, or at least your attitude towards it, may be determined to some extent at least by your own experience of childhood, and for some of you, your own experience of being parents or grandparents. For some, a positive childhood experience will strengthen a commitment to ensuring that others have this too. For others, a negative childhood experience may strengthen a resolve to help make it better for others. There are many excellent social workers and other professionals working with children who themselves have been previous victims of abuse. But they have subsequently sought appropriate help to ensure that these experiences do not get in the way of their work, but rather deepen their motivation to protect others from similar harm. Some adults find children a bit 'scary', especially when they enter their teenage years: they feel that they do not know how to talk with them, and find their 'grunt-laden apathy' or their boundary-testing exuberance too hot to handle. Others, by contrast, exult in the freshness, enthusiasm and uncertainties of teenagers, and get a huge buzz from working with them. Furthermore, your experiences of your school days are as varied as they could possibly be, and these too will have had some impact upon how you view young people currently going through a school education.

Exercise 3

The previous paragraph touched on different attitudes to children and young people, and how your experiences may impact upon your approach. This exercise is intended to help you 'locate yourself' as a worker, and to help you understand yourself a bit better. Make two lists on a piece of paper: the first list is all the positive experiences and memories of being a child and a young person that you can recall; the second is a list of all the negative, difficult and painful memories and experiences you can recall. Be as honest as you can, and try not to rush the exercise. When you have completed it, think about what are the implications for you in your work with children. It would be good to share this list with someone you can trust, and if you are a student in training it would be good to use this as a basis for a super-vision session looking at your values and how you are approaching this kind of work. Keep the list safe – you may find you want to add to it as time goes by. Remember, the most important thing you bring to your work is yourself, and how you come across to people will deter-mine to a great extent how effective you can be as a worker.

Many of the core communication skills discussed in this dictionary are as relevant to working with children as they are to adults. People of all ages need to know that they are accepted and valued; they deserve to receive an anti-discriminatory service, and to feel that they are included in what is being done in a real partnership. Just because they are young in years does not mean that these core communication skills are any less relevant. They welcome positive feedback just as anyone else does, and will thrive on an empowering approach. The challenges of diversity remain just as acute: children and young people from minority ethnic groups, or who have learning difficulties, or some experience of disability need workers who are aware of the wider cultural and societal aspects to discrimination and oppression, and who can incorporate these perspectives appropriately into their practice. In short, children and young people deserve the same 'gold standard' service as anyone else in the community: anything less is a betrayal of the best practice commitment all people workers need to uphold.

The foundation document for making assessments for all children is, of course, the *Framework for the Assessment of Children in Need and their Families* (2000), but there is additional guidance for working with disabled children in *Assessing Children in Need and their Families: Practice Guidance* (DoH, 2000). It is important that you are familiar with these documents and the information and guidance that they contain.

Harrison and Wise (2005: 40) provide a useful list of the communication skills necessary for the safeguarding and promoting of the welfare of the child. These include:

- establish rapport and respectful, trusting relationships with children, young people and those caring for them
- understand what is meant by safeguarding and the different ways in which children and young people can be harmed (including by other children and young people and through the Internet)
- make considered judgments about how to safeguard and promote a child or young person's welfare, and where appropriate consult with the child, young person, parent or carer to inform your thinking
- give the child or young person the opportunity to participate in decisions affecting them, as appropriate to their age and ability, and taking their wishes and feelings into account
- understand the key role of parents and carers in safeguarding and promoting children and young people's welfare and involve them accordingly, while recognising factors that can affect parenting and increase the risk of abuse (for example, domestic violence)
- understand that signs of abuse can be subtle and be expressed in play, artwork and in the way children and young people approach relationships with other children and/or adults
- make considered judgments about how to act to safeguard and promote a child or young person's welfare
- give the child or young person the opportunity to participate in decisions affecting them, as appropriate to their age and ability (pp. 33–34)
- be able to use clear language to communicate information unambiguously to others including children, young people, their families and carers
- listen carefully to what is said and check understanding.

Exercise 4

Spend some time working through the list of communication skills given above, and identify those areas where you feel you would need particular help and support in being able to achieve a successful outcome. You may find it helpful to have a particular example in mind of some work you have done to help you focus on these issues. Take the outcome of your reflections to supervision for more detailed discussion and guidance.

Complex needs

It is perhaps in working with disabled children, and children with complex needs, that the range of communication skills becomes somewhat widened. It is important of course to stress that in whatever professional capacity you work, there is a network of support and supervision that is crucial for you to learn about, practise, and gain competence in using the appropriate communication skills. You should not be thrown in at the deep end or left to flounder; there is considerable professional expertise upon which you can draw to develop your own skills.

It will be clear to you that when it comes to definitions, the notion of complex needs is very wide ranging, but generally it refers to children who have more than one impairment, or who have major health care needs such as life-limiting conditions, and those who have developed an impairment as a result of maltreatment or abuse. The communication skills you will need to develop, therefore, must be appropriate to the specific needs of the individual child. There is always a danger of compartmentalising such needs, of course, and you are advised to consult specialist literature and relevant colleagues to help you work with particular children with complex needs.

It is important, however, that you now return to the point made at the outset of this discussion. You need to be aware of the impact of such issues upon you, your attitudes, values and approach. Some children with complex needs present the worker with particular challenges, especially if there is physical disfigurement, or uncoordinated speech or physical movement. As a worker you need to be aware of the impact of your non-verbal communication towards the young person and the family: if you feel an element of revulsion (this is a strong word to use, but there is no point in pussyfooting around such issues, which can provoke strong reactions in some people) then this will communicate itself very clearly to them. It is of vital importance, therefore, that you examine your own value-base and your own attitudes in advance of such work, so that you can ensure that you provide the level of acceptance, respect and care that the person has every right to receive from you. This is part of what is mean by being a reflective practitioner.

You will have noticed throughout this entire discussion that you as a worker are being put in the spotlight, as far as communication skills are concerned, far more than the particular child or young person who has complex needs. This is not to minimise the child's needs or the quality of complex services that may be necessary. On the contrary. But it does emphasis the importance of you as the worker, *what* you are communicating and *how* you are communicating. If you can get that right, the other things will follow, given appropriate support, advice, training and guidance.

Final thoughts

Anyone working with children and young people will be aware of the vast literature that now exists to encourage, support and guide workers in this important field, both for generic working and for the delivery of more specialist services. A few of these are listed below, but within your agency you will have access to much more.

References and Further reading

Aldridge, M. and Wood, J. (1998) *Interviewing Children. A Guide for Child Care and Forensic Practitioners*. Chichester: Wiley.

Department of Health (2000) *Framework for the Assessment of Children in Need and Their Families*. London: The Stationery Office.

Department of Health (2000) *Assessing Children in Need and Their Families: Practice Guidance*. London: The Stationery Office.

DfES (2004) *Every Child Matters*. London: DfES.

Harrison, R. and Wise, C. (2005) *Working with Young People*. London: Sage.

Home Office (1992) *Memorandum of Good Practice*. London: The Stationery Office.

Jowitt, M. and O'Loughlin, S. (2005) *Social Work with Children and Families*. Exeter: Learning Matters.

Social Care Institute for Excellence (SCIE) (2006) *Teaching, Learning and Assessing Communication Skills with Children and Young People in Social Work Education*. London: Social Care Institute for Excellence.

Related concepts Acceptance; anti-discriminatory practice; assessment; empowerment; feedback; non-verbal communication; partnership; reflective practice.

Learning Difficulties

An entry on learning difficulties in a dictionary of communication skills immediately risks causing some disquiet. There is the risk of assuming a 'them and us' mentality, whereby we mistakenly attribute all sorts of communication problems to one group of people who somehow are not as fortunate as other groups of people. People with learning difficulties (or disabilities: the language used is notoriously slippery) are often lumped together in very discriminatory and oppressive ways, not only by the general public, but also at times by professional people-workers. The term 'learning difficulty' is often to be preferred because it conveys the message that certain things about being human and getting on with living and loving, are found to be difficult. And there is no one alive who cannot identify to some extent with that statement!

The first point to stress, therefore, is the value-base that underpins all people-work. The importance of affording acceptance, dignity, respect and value to each and every human being is a principle that is non-negotiable. Therefore the communication skills, both verbal and non-verbal, that both embody and reflect these principles should be the same for everyone, no matter what additional labels they may be given. The Government White Paper 'Valuing People' (2001) seeks to embody and 'flesh out' what a value-based approach to work with people with learning difficulties might look like.

A second introductory and underpinning point stresses the talents, gifts, creative abilities and resilience that we believe everyone has to a greater or lesser extent. Therefore, the basic principles of partnership-working, empowerment and the clutch of issues that are raised by an awareness of people's spirituality are all not only relevant, but crucial to our approach. We must always be open to being caught by surprise when another person's talents burst forth in unexpected ways and places. It is to our shame that often we do not expect people with learning difficulties to surprise us, even though, as Williams (2006: 120) notes:

> There are people so described who have written poetry and books, become accomplished artists and performers, given talks at conference, have

played a valuable role in teaching professionals, have acted as consultants on government policy and so on.

The third point to make is that we often talk as if all the problems and difficulties lie with the other person, not ourselves. But time and time again the real problem may lie just as much with us, and our inability to understand, reach out, and empathise. Just as it always takes two to tango, it takes two to communicate; and if you are putting up barriers, then is it surprising that communication is difficult?

Exercise 1

Spend some time reflecting on the three introductory points made above, and relate them to any people with learning difficulties you know. Have you discovered in yourself the temptation to play down these core values in your dealings with them? What do you feel are the biggest issues for you in seeking to establish meaningful and effective communication with people with learning difficulties?

If you have completed this exercise honestly, a number of reactions may have been triggered off for you. You may have been able to acknowledge, for example, some aspects of learning difficulty within yourself. Most, if not all of us struggle to learn certain skills, or to express ourselves clearly, and a realistic awareness of this, tinged with a degree of humility, can help to reinforce the bonds of common humanity between us and those with whom we are called to work in our professional people-work roles.

Another reaction may be elicited by certain physical characteristics in others that you may find disturbing. The key issue here is captured in the words *that you may find disturbing*. This indicates that the problem, if indeed there is a problem, lies with you and your inability or unwillingness really to celebrate diversity. Other people's difference will have an impact upon you and how you relate to them. And as the discussion on non-verbal communication reveals, these deep feelings will communicate themselves to others very easily. If you feel embarrassed or disgusted, that will communicate itself to the other person, and will counteract any words you use that are intended to convey your professional value-base of acceptance and respect. The importance of reflective practice, therefore, cannot be underestimated.

Within this overall framework of values that underpin your professional practice, there are some communication skills, however, that are particularly appropriate to use with people with very severe impairments. Two systems are often found to be helpful: Makaton and Signalong, which are simplifed variations of British Sign Language, which is the principal and very fluent first language of the Deaf community. Another approach is the use of the 'widgit' system that enables written words to be turned into visual symbols. These systems can be enormously helpful aids to communication, but clearly they need a mutual familiarity for them to be effective, and a sensitive, patient approach by the worker (for further details of these three systems see www.makaton.org; www.signalong.org.uk; www.widget.co.uk).

There is a temptation, however, to try to shoe-horn everyone into a handful of communication 'techniques', and to assume that one size fits all. The real communication skill, though, lies in seeking out what is most effective for each individual. Some people, for example, thrive on the possibilities of new electronic technologies that can enable people, who previously had been unable to express themselves clearly to others, to begin to pour their self-expression onto the screen. 'Facilitated communication', whereby someone guides and supports the other person to help them write and spell words, has also had some dramatic creative results (see Williams, 2006: 122, for some examples). For others, more basic approaches are preferred.

Key points to bear in mind when seeking to communicate with someone with learning difficulties include the following:

- remember that the other person is the 'expert' and will know what works best; each person is unique
- key principles of acceptance, dignity, respect and working in partnership must always be central to your approach
- your own non-verbal communication skills will be particularly important
- be reflective in trying to identify, and then remove barriers you are putting up that get in the way of effective communication
- a trusting relationship is crucial – however mechanistic a 'system' such as Makaton may seem, it is the quality of your relationship that is all important
- explore ways of helping the other person to 'play to their strengths'
- work in partnership with others who may know the other person far better than you do.

Final thoughts

The stories you hear about the ways in which people with learning difficulties are sometimes treated – stories of abuse, of not being treated with respect and dignity, or being refused entry to restaurants, for example – will remind you that underlying all communication skills is your value-base. Until you get that right, you will not be able really to communicate appropriately with another human being, nor treat them with dignity and respect.

References and Further reading

Swinton, J. (2002) 'Spirituality and the lives of people with learning disabilities', *The Tizard Learning Disability Review,* 7(4): 29–35.
Williams, P. (2006) *Social Work with People with Learning Difficulties.* Exeter: Learning Matters. (NB: this book has much to offer people-workers from other disciplines)

Related concepts   Active listening skills; non-verbal communication; partnership working; reflective practice; spirituality.

Loss

The experience of loss is one of the common themes running through a wide range of people-work: dealing with loss is a cost of being human. It is, therefore, important that people-workers develop the communication skills to be able sensitively and appropriately to work with people who are experiencing loss.

Exercise 1

Jot down as many examples of loss as you can think of. Include minor losses as well as major ones. Keep this list beside you as you work through this discussion.

The list you have just compiled may well grow in length the more you think about it. It is likely that you will have included some of the major losses, such as divorce, unemployment, ill health and bereavement, as well as a wide variety of seemingly less significant losses, like losing your watch or a favourite item of clothing. Some losses are difficult to define, such as the loss of faith or confidence, while others may be too painful to share with other people.

In thinking about the communication skills needed to work with people experiencing loss, it is important to acknowledge that perhaps more than any other topic, this can deeply affect us as workers. Because the experience of loss is so pervasive, we too will have our own experiences of it, and in some ways how we have dealt with loss will have some impact upon how we respond to others going through a similar experience. For example:

- If you have not fully grieved over the loss of someone close to you, you may find that working with someone recently and painfully bereaved can trigger painful memories within you which you desperately want to ignore or run away from.
- If you have had a difficult or painful experience of divorce within your own family, you may find that working with couples with children who are separating extremely upsetting.
- If in the past you have been 'given the sack' from a job and are trying to work with a person in a similar situation, you may find yourself strongly identifying with them and assuming that what was true for you will be true for them. You may find yourself urging them to pursue a course of action that seems right to you, based on your experience, but which may not be right for them.
- If your own experiences of loss are difficult and painful you may find yourself steering conversations and interviews away from this topic in order to make the interview more manageable and bearable for you, even if the other person really needs to discuss it.

These examples illustrate how a negative experience can negatively affect your working relationship with others if you are not careful. By contrast, however, if you have yourself been 'through the prickly hedge of grief and loss', and know what it is to be supported and cared for in a positive way and have benefitted from this, then you are more likely to be open to exploring this area with others, and to offering the kind of support which you know will most likely to be effective and appreciated.

Exercise 2

Spend a few moments thinking about an experience of loss in your own life. How did you feel? How did others respond to you? Can you identify some responses which you found really helpful, and others which 'made your toes curl', making you angry and resentful?

This emphasis upon our experience of loss as workers is important, because inevitably we will be communicating to the other person non-verbally a number of messages which they will pick up even more quickly because of the rawness and sensitivity of their own feelings. So, if you are feeling awkward, embarrassed, tense, agitated or scared, this will communicate itself to the other person who will perhaps think twice before opening up about how they are really feeling. If, on the other hand, you can convey warmth, acceptance, a sense of stillness and a willingness to be with the other person, then it is likely that they will pick up the message that it is OK and safe to talk to you, because somehow, just somehow, you may understand.

In other words, how we deal with our own losses will determine to a large extent how we deal with others in their loss.

The second main area for us as people-workers to grasp when developing our communication skills going through times of loss, is the importance of a sound theoretical perspective to help us – and the other person – understand what they are going through. There are several dimensions to this.

1 The person who is experiencing the loss is the only one who can say how intense their feelings are. What may seem to the worker to be a minor loss, such as the death of a pet budgerigar, for example, may be a major loss to the older person who had been living alone unable to get out and about, and for whom the budgie was a real source of comfort and company, and even perhaps a reason to keep going. If the worker seeks to minimise the impact of a loss, this could be a cause of great resentment by the other person, who will immediately draw the conclusion that the worker simply does not understand.

2 Comforting words are often not comforting. Workers can easily fall into the trap of thinking that there is a word for every occasion, and seek to offer comfort with what are often no more than platitudes. For example:

- You'll soon get over it.
- There are plenty of other fish in the sea.
- You'll be OK, I promise.
- There are plenty of others worse than you.
- Try to pull yourself together.
- Why don't you take up a hobby, get out and meet people.

There is, of course, a tiny germ of truth lurking in each of these statements, and they are often made with the best will in the world, but they rarely help: they tell us more about the worker than the person going through the pain of grief; they tell us more about where the worker is coming from than where the other person is currently standing. At best they are well meaning; at worst, they are a banal 'whistling in the dark' by a bemused worker who does not know how to communicate with someone experiencing loss.

3   There is no automatic process for dealing with grief and loss. Many people-workers have been brought up on the seminal work by Elizabeth Kubler Ross (1969), who, with others, talked about the stages of grief through which people need to pass before reaching the final point of acceptance. Her work with dying people revealed some of the profound feelings that loss provokes: shock, anger, denial, despair. Anyone who has experienced a profound loss will identify with these feelings, and know how powerful they can be. What has been less helpful is the way in which some people-workers have used this model of stages almost to predict the journey through grief, and to regard the model as being prescriptive. A lot of contemporary theorists have helped us move towards a more complex and realistic understanding of how people respond to grief and loss, by reminding us that everyone's journey is unique, and we each of us choose, consciously or otherwise, how we will handle such matters. Two contemporary approaches may be of particular help to people-workers in general.

Neimeyer (2001) talks about meaning reconstruction, which emphasises that it is the person who is experiencing the grief and loss who knows the *meaning* of that loss, and more importantly how new meanings will need to be created if life is to go on in any meaningful way in the future. This journey towards new meanings may be never-ending of course, but the search for them is critical.

The 'dual process' model of Stroebe and Schutt (1999) talks of two orientations when we experience loss: the past and the present/future. The journey of grief will see people moving in and out of these two orientations, sometimes many times in a day, as they are at one time overwhelmed by the loss, and at other times facing the daily tasks which have to be done, while looking ahead. As time goes by they will spend less and less time in the past orientation, but it will never go away, and is likely to be re-stimulated at key moments in a year, such as anniversaries, or by key moments such as hearing a particular tune or going to a particular place.

This is but a quick snapshot of some of the theoretical perspectives which are enriching our understanding of grief and loss, and you are encouraged to explore these in greater depth, together with other perspectives, through the further reading. The perspectives that have been covered, however, are sufficient to illustrate some of the main communication skills necessary when working with people who are experiencing loss. These include:

- **Non-verbal communication** Be open, accepting and unhurried in your approach – do not sit with arms crossed or look as if you have chewed a wasp; avoid barrier gestures; watch with smiling eyes and a subtle, warm but not cheery smile.
- **Ask don't tell** Invite the person to say how they are feeling, and what their loss means to them. Encourage them to talk about their loss if they wish.
- **Explain but don't predict** Your grasp of theoretical perspectives and how people often react to serious loss can be helpful to others if you handle things sensitively. The dual process model, for example, can be explained simply to reassure people that they will ebb and flow in their feelings, probably for quite a long time, and this is not something to be unduly worried about. The more precious something or someone has been to them, the more acute and long-lasting the reactions to the loss will be. Maybe they will never ever fully 'get over' the loss or come to terms with it: in such situations their future may be about learning to surround the gaping hole in their lives with various people and activities, knowing full well that the hole will never close. The thing to avoid is predicting how people will react: we are all different and we cannot predict when or how people will deal with their loss. If, for example, as sometimes happen, workers slavishly follow the stages model and try to reassure people that after such-and-such a stage things will improve, this could be disheartening for the person if this is not how it turns out for them. It sometimes happens that people who have heard of the stages model feel that they are doing something wrong when things do not follow the pattern they have been led to expect. Again, the reassurance lies in explaining to people that we all do things differently, and that getting it right for them is the crucial thing. It can help sometimes to explain to people that a certain range of feelings is common, that a loss of energy or interest is to be expected, and that physical symptoms such as backache can sometimes be experienced; it is not unusual for some people to feel that they are in a dark tunnel that has no end to it. Again, tempting though it is to try to predict how soon these feelings will abate, we cannot do this with any integrity: after all, we could be very wrong in our predictions. Instead, finding ways of empathising with their pain, fear and discomfort is far more helpful in the long run.
- **Share their journey; don't make it your own** The discussion on empathy is helpful here. What people seem to find helpful is not

to hear all about the worker's similar experiences or how other people have coped (or not), but to have someone who will listen in a caring non-judgmental way, to help them feel at least to a small extent that they are not as totally alone as they had feared. We can never fully understand or get inside another person's experience of loss, or what it means to them, but if we make the attempt it can prove to be very supportive. But we must not make the other person's burden our own, or get so embroiled in their difficulties that we lose our objectivity and professional distance. This is why an awareness of our own losses is so important: if the other person's loss triggers off painful deep-seated feelings within us, then we begin to lose our professional perspective and become part of the problem rather than providing support to the person on their journey.

- **Explore; don't interrogate** The style you adopt in talking with someone experiencing loss is all important. Too vigorous, insensitive or persistent questioning will likely make someone 'close down' and become resentful: it will feel that their personal space is being invaded. You can, however, begin to explore with the person how they think they will begin to face and re-shape their future, and begin to engage with the meaning re-construction that will soon be necessary, to a greater or lesser extent. But if you push too hard and give the impression that you are expecting the other person to come up with clear-cut answers and strategies, then you are likely to undermine what little confidence they have clung onto.

  The issue of people's religious faith, or their more general spirituality which shapes their world-view, is another issue that needs sometimes to be explored in an open, sensitive way. In all cases, as the worker you must ensure that whatever is the world-view to which you personally subscribe, it is the other person's world-view that is important and the extent to which it proves satisfying and helpful in moments of crisis and loss.

Final thoughts

Because loss is such a pervasive experience, it is inevitable that it will directly impinge upon every practitioner from time to time with the people who come to them. The general guidelines for the range of communication skills you need to be able to exercise will stand you in good stead, and help to ensure that the person feels valued and supported. However, there may well be situations where the other person seems so deeply immersed, even trapped, in their feelings of loss, pain and disempowerment that you realise that they need more specific professional help than you are able to provide. In such situations you need to know what range of local services, including bereavement counselling, is available, and to find sensitive ways of referring people to these services without seeming to reject them. It is important that you feel able to use the general communication skills guidelines we have suggested here, but it is also vital that you know your limitations and do not try to swim in waters that are far too deep for you to navigate successfully and professionally.

Reference and Further reading

Kubler Ross, E. (1969) *On Death and Dying*. New York: Macmillan.

Leming, M. and Dickinson, G. (2002) *Understanding Death, Dying and Bereavement*. 5th edition. Orlando, Fl.: Harcourt College Publishers.

Moss, B. (2004) *Working with Loss: A Training Resource Pack for Human Service Practitioners*. Wrexham: Learning Curve Publications.

Moss, B. (2005) *Religion and Spirituality*. Lyme Regis: Russell House Publishing.

Neimeyer, R. (2001) *Meaning Reconstruction and the Meaning of Loss*. Washington DC: American Psychological Association.

Stroebe, M. and Schutt, M. (1999) 'The dual process model of coping with bereavement: rationale and description', *Death Studies*, 23(3): 197–224.

Thompson, N. (2002) *Loss and Grief: A Guide for Human Services Practitioners*. Basingstoke: Palgrave.

Related concepts   Active listening; barrier gestures; empathy; non-verbal communication; religion; spirituality.

Mediation Skills

Mediation, as a practice discipline, is a very skilled process whereby a person 'in the middle' seeks to facilitate a creative, acceptable outcome for two people who are in dispute and conflict with each other. The person in the middle – the mediator – seeks impartially to create an environment of mutual respect to enable the disputants to come to some level of agreement, thereby enabling them to move forward. This process, sometimes also referred to as Alternative Dispute Resolution (ADR), is becoming increasingly popular in a wide range of settings, not least since Lord Justice Wolfe's report (1995; 1996) recommended its use in many legal disputes as an alternative to litigation.

It is important at the outset to say that social workers, advice workers, and the various people-workers who seek to offer help, support, guidance and advice to people in a variety of needs are not mediators in the strictest sense. Mediation as a discrete service is available to people who wish, or need to avail themselves of it. By including mediation in this book, however, it is not being suggested that the community has a far wider army of mediators than is immediately apparent. Unfortunately some areas in the country still do not have easy access to such services.

What is being suggested, however, is that mediation *skills* are much more generic, and are enormously important elements in your bag of skills. This is because these skills are central in dealing effectively with conflict, and conflict is at the heart of a lot of people-work, no matter what agency you work for.

This is not to assume that all conflict is necessarily bad. On the contrary, whenever we seek to change the way in which we, and others around us, behave, conflict is inevitable; all sorts of good changes and positive advances will involve a measure of conflict in order to effect positive change. The problems occur when the effect of conflict is negative; when people get stuck and refuse to budge, and begin to take up positions that they will defend at all costs. Mediation skills are useful for defusing negative conflict, helping people to 'unhook' themselves from fixed positions, and releasing a vision of what the future might be like if the conflict could be resolved creatively.

It would be wrong to assume that situations of conflict will only occur between people who use your services or whose relationships have seriously deteriorated. Some of the most debilitating conflicts for people-workers can be internal to their agency, where clashes of opinion or personality can make a team an unhappy and unproductive place to work. Managers often have to take difficult decisions about resource allocations, leading workers sometimes to feel that they have returned to the era of the 'deserving' and 'undeserving' poor.

Some conflicts, of course, are unresolvable, especially when you are trying to make finite resources stretch to meet seemingly infinite need, or where people simply will not budge or give way. Some people enjoy a good conflict or battle, just as some people seem to need to have their day in court and to hand over the ultimate decision about the outcome of their dispute to someone else, preferably a person in authority like a magistrate or judge, or an arbitrator. Some divorcing parents choose to have their residence and contact disputes decided by a court because one or other of the parents does not want to appear to their children to be giving up their parenting claim, and prefer to leave the decision for a wise judge to make.

These examples are at the extreme end of the spectrum of course, and in your everyday work you are more likely to come across less serious examples of conflict, where you could well make a considerable impact by a judicious use of mediation skills.

But before we explore these, here is an exercise to help you provide a context for the discussion that follows.

Exercise 1

Think of two or three examples of conflict you have experienced recently, where people have been in dispute. If you can, try to recall something which involves the people who come to you for help, and then something involving the team in which you are currently working. Make a few notes on the following questions:

- What was the conflict about?
- What were the key issues involved?
- Why do you think they seemed unable to achieve an amicable outcome?

Even though in a strict sense you may not be acting as a mediator, nevertheless, you may well find that by carefully using some mediation skills you are able to facilitate a good outcome. Although many of these skills are generic and useful to any type of people work, some are claimed by mediators to be specific to their dispute resolution role.

The range of skills includes:

Active listening and clarifying   This goes without saying, perhaps, but unless you are able to listen really carefully, you will not be able to make much progress. Listening is not just about hearing and understanding what those in dispute are saying to each other; it is also about listening for what each of them is *not* saying, the issues they are *not* raising. These are the issues which are often at the heart of the conflict, because they indicate what each of the parties is frightened about. Conflicts often occur when people's interests are threatened or undermined in some way; they can get very defensive and aggressive at the prospect of losing out in some way. It is important to note that such fears may be well founded, or at times completely irrational. Active listening will attempt to identify what the conflict is about; what the key issues are, and what is preventing them from reaching an amicable solution.

Active listening is also a visual activity, whereby you pick up what are often called the 'non-verbal signals' which each of the disputants is giving out. How people look at each other; what hand gestures they make; how they sit; how they respond physically to what is being said or alleged – all reveal important information about what is going on inside each person and how they are feeling. At times the non-verbal signals can contradict the words people use, and nine times out of ten it will be the non-verbal signals which reveal what the person is *really* trying to communicate.

Another feature of active listening within the context of a dispute is the skill of interpreting and clarifying what is being said. People in dispute do not always think clearly when they are under pressure; sentences sometimes come tumbling out in the heat of the moment that, on reflection, they would have preferred to say differently. Sometimes words seem very inadequate tools to use to convey meaning fully. And when people are in the turbulence of an argument or dispute, there is no guarantee that each will hear clearly what the other is saying. Indeed, it is more than likely that on occasion they will seize on one aspect of what is being said to them, and ignore the rest. We all can get hold of the wrong end of the stick, and in disputes sticks often seem to have more wrong ends than we would ever realise!

An important listening and communication skill, therefore, for someone who is 'in the middle' is to look for occasions when mis-hearing or mis-communication is taking place. There is an important role for you to play, in checking out with those concerned whether that was really what they intended to say, or whether they had really intended this or that interpretation to be given to what was said. Sometimes the simple process of clarifying, and asking whether or not 'this or that' was what the person really intended, can play an important part in enabling people in dispute to begin to listen to each other, rather than talk past each other. By undertaking this clarifying role, which may involve the use of a range of questions to each of them, you may well find that people who have appeared not to be able to 'see the wood for the trees' begin to understand each other better. This is often the first step towards a resolution.

Summarising   This is an important communication skill to use if you are seeking to help resolve a dispute. In the early stages of an argument there may often be 'more heat than light', and from time to time it will be important for you to take some control of what is happening and reflect back to each of the people how you see the story so far. This skill of summarising can serve a number of purposes:

- It reminds people that you are trying to play a role in helping them to come to a solution.
- It can take the heat out of the situation, even if only briefly.
- It provides each of them an opportunity to look into a mirror and to see what impression they have been creating to an outsider.
- It provides them with an opportunity to hear themselves and what they have been saying. Rather like hearing a tape recording, they can check whether what you are reflecting back to them is really what they intend to say or not. It does not matter too much whether you have got it completely right: if you have missed something, or got something wrong, they will be quick to point this out, and this will in itself aid further clarification.
- It provides an opportunity to decide on what the steps are to be in seeking a resolution.

Mutualising, normalising and re-framing   These skills are sometimes claimed to be unique to the mediation process, but they have a more general application. 'Mutualising' is a communication skill that seeks to recognise common ground between the people in dispute. It can help them realise that, far from being poles apart, they may be closer to coming to a solution than they had realised. If you can demonstrate the common concerns and interests they share, it can often help people move forward. A classic example of this is when divorcing parents argue, sometimes bitterly, about what is best for their children. A mutualising statement would acknowledge that each of them as parents really loves the children and wants what is best for them.

Normalising is a skill that you can use to help people pull back from the brink in a dispute. Because we are human, we often tend to assume that the problems we encounter are so unique to us that they are in a different league from anyone else's. In one sense, of course, that is perfectly true: there is only one of us in the whole world and how we experience things will be unique to us. But the temptation when we are in a dispute is to ratchet up this claim to uniqueness, and to give the impression *that the problems and issues that we are raising are so different from anything else anyone else has ever experienced that it will be 'beyond the wit' of anyone to come up with a decent solution.* In other words, we place ourselves in what we believe is a safe place where only a 100 per cent capitulation by the other person will be enough.

However, the experience of mediators and of other helping professionals is that the sort of difficulties people experience do have common themes or strands to them. Many people who experience similar problems in fact have worked at it and have come up with perfectly acceptable solutions. Sometimes people need reassuring that the feelings which at times overwhelm them when they are in dispute often go with the territory, and need not block a solution being found.

Re-framing is a skill that can be very effective for you to use if you are trying to help people resolve a conflict. It is natural for people in a dispute to want to tell their own story from their own point of view. They will view events, and relate them to you and to the person they are in conflict with, through one particular lens. This is not necessarily a case of wearing 'rose tinted spectacles', but it will be an example of looking at the situation from one particular point of view. It is often the case that one person's perception will ensure that the other person is seen in a negative light. If, in your role as the middle person in the dispute, you can suggest other, more positive ways of looking at a situation, then you will be trying to 're-frame'. The previous example of two parents in dispute over their children would be a good example of this. If the mediator were to take a complaint about one parent's behaviour towards the children, and help the other person see that what really is motivating them is a desire to be a good parent, then this would be an example of positive re-framing. It could well then lead on to a mutual acknowledgement that both of them have the best interests of their children at heart.

Looking towards a 'win–win' outcome   Although there are sometimes conflicts and disputes where one person is clearly in the wrong, and the decision has to go in favour of the other person, in many arguments and disputes it is more likely that what is needed is a solution to which both of them can subscribe, and feel committed towards making it work in practice. If one person 'wins hands down', the person who loses will feel demoralised, de-motivated and perhaps even humiliated. The best solutions, therefore, will be the ones where each person can walk away feeling that they *had* fully expressed their concerns and points of view, and *had* come to a working solution which they are able to accept. This is clearly going to be important where people still need to work or live together. It is a skill, therefore, that anyone seeking to help resolve conflict needs to keep clearly in focus.

Exercise 2

Return to the scenarios you identified in Exercise 1, and explore how you might be able to use some of the skills outlined above in helping to work towards a resolution.

Final thoughts

No one pretends that you will find these skills easy to practise. At times you will feel drawn more towards one side of the conflict than the other, and the temptation to take sides will be strong. Your own experiences of conflict and how you feel about them, how you have emerged from disputes, and what you feel about conflict will all play a part in how you behave when caught up in a mediating role with people who are in dispute. Sometimes to hold the middle ground is the hardest task of all, but if you are to be effective in seeking to help people resolve their conflict, it is the only place to be.

References and Further reading

Brown, H. and Marriott, A. (1999) *ADR Principles and Practice.*
    2nd edition. London: Sweet & Maxwell.
Charlton, R. and Dewdney, M. (2004) *The Mediator's Handbook.*
    2nd edition. Sydney: Lawbook Co.
Stewart, S. (1998) *Conflict Resolution: A Foundation Guide.*
    Winchester: Waterside Press.
Taylor, M. (2005) *Negotiation.* Inns of Court School of Law.
    Oxford: Oxford University Press.
Wolfe, L.J. (1995, 1996) Interim report to the Lord Chancellor on
    the Civil Justice system in England and Wales 1995; and
    Access to Justice, July 1996.

Related concepts   Active listening; conflict management; non-verbal communication.

Non-verbal Communication

It is often said that a picture is worth a thousand words. By this is meant that a picture can convey in breadth and depth a far wider and more complex set of meanings in its constricted space on the canvas than would be possible by just using words alone. This is not meant to diminish the power of words; rather, it paints for us a wider context in which communication takes place.

If, for a moment, we regard our physical body as a picture that we are presenting to the people with whom we work, then a similar point can be made. What we communicate to that person is more than the actual words we use: it is the whole bundle of messages, signals and symbols that our physical presence conveys. Whatever words a police officer or traffic warden may use when challenging us with a misdemeanour, it will be the symbol of their uniform that makes the greatest impact upon us. This conveys the very clear message: *mess with me at your peril.*

In her discussion of non-verbal communication, Trevithick (2005: 120) refers to a study by Birdwhistell (1970) which demonstrated that:

> in a typical encounter involving two people, the actual spoken or verbal content is likely to carry only one third of the social meaning in any given encounter, whereas the non-verbal forms convey roughly two thirds of the meaning. In addition, it is estimated that more weight is given to non-verbal forms of communication ...

This has profound implications for anyone involved in people-work. It is not saying that the words we use are unimportant – far from it. But it is suggesting that our words are only some of the paints we use to produce the picture of our interaction with someone, and that non-verbal communication skills are likely to be far more dominant, and have a far greater impact overall.

Some examples will help to illustrate the point:

- You are sitting with someone who has recently been bereaved. There is nothing you can say to alleviate their distress, but you sit quietly and allow them to talk or cry, or to be silent. When you leave you are surprised to hear them say to you how much they have appreciated your visit and how helpful it has been.

- A social worker goes to court to present a report on a young person, and turns up dressed in a sloppy pullover and jeans, and is asked by the magistrates to leave the court.
- A female worker in a male bail hostel turns up to help run a group-work session wearing a low-cut FCUK top and a mini skirt, and is asked by the manager to go home and come back dressed more appropriately.
- A community worker arrives to visit a family who have massive debt problems and a range of other difficulties, dressed in a sharp expensive suit, gold cufflinks, and carrying an expensive leather briefcase, and is surprised by the cold reception he receives.

Exercise 1

Identify and discuss the four scenarios outlined above. What do you think are the key issues with each of them in terms of non-verbal communication? Do you agree with the decisions taken in the second and third scenarios?

These scenarios illustrate the point that, in each case, the person involved was communicating a very powerful message about themselves non-verbally, which was picked up and responded to. It is important to note that these examples – and indeed this whole discussion – are focusing only on non-verbal communication in a professional or work-based setting, and the roles that we fulfil.

Non-verbal communication through how we dress or behave is also an issue in our personal and social lives, but there are different issues involved there which are not quite so relevant to this discussion. Nevertheless, it has to be said that whether in a professional or personal context the way a person dresses should never be regarded as an invitation to any advances or behaviour that is deemed unacceptable or threatening to the person concerned.

Before going into more detail, it is important to stress that we do have control over our non-verbal communication, and that it can rightly be regarded as a communication skill. How we dress says something very important to the people with whom we come into contact. The various settings you become involved in have a significant impact upon how you dress and present yourselves. You need to give some thought to this. To turn up in a formal setting, such as court, shabbily dressed is not only going to be regarded as disrespectful to the court, it also runs the risk of doing a major disservice to the person you are seeking to represent or support. A 'take it or leave it' or 'this is not something to get worked up about' approach, conveyed by the casual attire, is not the message the court expects you to give.

It is important to recognise the *context* of your work with people, and the non-verbal messages which can be conveyed. For example, you are conveying non-verbal messages in all of the following ways:

- whether you are punctual for your appointments, and keep to the time allotted for your visit or interview
- how you dress and the appearance you present to people
- how you arrange the room if you are meeting people at the office
- whether you offer a symbolic touch to people, such as a handshake
- how you manage the space or distance between yourself and the other person
- whether you offer refreshments to people
- how you sit; your posture, and how you move; whether or not you fidget
- whether or not you smile; your facial expressions and gestures
- how you bring the meeting to a close and take your leave.

There are other non-verbal aspects of communication that can be important from time to time. For example:

- When you visit a person in their own home, wait to be shown where they would like you to sit; allow a pause for them to clear away any clutter.
- If there are dogs in the house and you are fearful of them, wait at the door until the dog is taken into another room.
- If the television is on and it is difficult to hear what is being said and you feel awkward about asking for it to be turned down, try moving your face closer to the person who is speaking, and glance at the TV – maybe point at the TV, and make a minimising gesture with your hand to invite it to be turned down or off. (Of course, if you feel able to ask them directly to turn it down or off, then this can be so much easier!)
- Make a point of switching your mobile phone onto silent or vibrate mode in front of the other person. This tells them that you are giving them undivided time, but also makes it clear that you can make a call if you need help or assistance.
- If you have any uncertainty about the person you are interviewing, ensure that you have an easy exit route by placing yourself near to the door.

So far we have concentrated on the skills that you need to develop across a wide range of non-verbal communication, and we have suggested that careful attention to these will help to ensure a much more successful outcome to your meetings or interviews. Certainly, if there is congruence between the non-verbal and verbal content of your interview, you will have been pretty effective in the task you have had to complete. By contrast, if the non-verbal signs and signals have contradicted what you have said, the 'non-verbals' will win 'hands down'.

Non-verbal communication also works in the other direction, of course, and you can tell a lot about the other person by 'reading the signs' accurately: how a person is dressed and how they present themselves, what their living conditions are like, how they greet you, how they hold themselves physically, how they respond to you; all these are signs and clues about how the other person is feeling, which can help you in your communication and assessment.

Non-verbal skills for handling aggression

One particularly difficult area where non-verbal communication is of central importance is in dealing with aggression. If someone becomes agitated, and starts jabbing a finger at you or waving a clenched fist, if they begin to raise their voice and start talking more quickly, or suddenly get up from their seat, you don't need much insight to realise that aggression is mounting, and that you may be at risk.

In extreme cases, your first priority must be for your own safety, and you may need to activate the panic button (if you are in the office context) or simply leave the room to seek help and escape the threat of violence.

There are, however, a number of non-verbal responses that you can use which may help to defuse the situation, even though quite understandably you will feel nervous, or afraid. A lot may depend, of course, on the gender mix of the interview: sometimes women can more easily defuse a situation when a man begins to show anger and aggression, but whatever the situation there are some guidelines that will prove helpful. These include:

- Try to remain calm, and breathe deeply.
- Stand up if the other person has stood up, but avoid adopting a confrontational posture.
- Ask the person by name to sit down; tell them that their behaviour makes it difficult for you to concentrate, and that you want to discuss what is bothering them.
- Speak and move a little more slowly than usual to help the other person slow down.
- Keep at a reasonable distance from the other person – out of arm's reach if possible.

159

- Do not attempt to touch the other person; keep your own hands and arms relaxed.
- Keep looking straight at the other person without staring, or smiling (this can sometimes be interpreted as mocking).
- Keep as still, relaxed and calm as possible.
- If you feel comfortable, sit down and invite the other person to sit so that you can resume your discussion.
- When things calm down a bit, ask if they would like a few minutes to collect their thoughts before you resume your discussion; would they like a drink (be careful though – you do not want hot cups of tea being thrown at you later on).

These are a few suggestions on how best to cope, and how to use non-verbal communication skills to defuse an aggressive situation. We repeat our initial advice, however: if you feel threatened and at risk, your first responsibility is to remove yourself from the situation as quickly as possible.

Exercise 2

It is always better to have discussed how you would handle such a situation with someone whom you feel you can trust, such as your supervisor or practice teacher. Your agency should have some clear guidelines and procedures as part of their health and safety policy, and you may well be able to undertake some role play with colleagues to help prepare you to deal with these situations.

Final thoughts

For people without speech, those who are Deaf or deafened, and those with specific communication difficulties, non-verbal communication is their main means of relating to other people. Many of the issues already raised in this discussion still remain relevant, but the principal means of communication will be different. British Sign Language (BSL), for example, is a language in its own right, celebrated and used by the Deaf community. It is a beautiful, 'liquid' flowing form of communication using fingers, hands and facial gestures. For Deaf/Blind people the language of BSL is communicated through touch. Makaton is an artificial system for basic communication that has been devised to help people without speech, or with limited verbal capacity, to communicate with others.

The advent of electronic and computer technology has enabled many people without speech to become far more fluent in their communication skills. Many disabled people can now use the computer to communicate even if they have limited or no manual dexterity. By using pointers which they can operate by mouth or as an attachment to their foreheads they are able to develop communication skills which have enhanced their quality of life.

References and Further reading

Birdwhistell, R. (1970) *Kinesics and Context*. Philadelphia, PA: University of Pennsylvania.
Koprowska, J. (2005) *Communication and Interpersonal Skills in Social Work*. Exeter: Learning Matters. (See chapter 9, Working with hostility)
Trevithick, P. (2005) *Social Work Skills: A Practice Handbook*. Maidenhead: Open University Press. (pp. 119 ff)
Williams, P. (2006) *Social Work with People with Learning Difficulties*. Exeter: Learning Matters.

Related concepts   Barrier gestures; conflict management; reflective practice.

Paraphrasing

(*see* active listening)

Partnership Working

(*see* assessment; empowerment)

Reflective Practice

In the Introduction you will have noted the emphasis that was laid upon reflective practice and its importance to your professional development. Two visual metaphorical images will help to make this point: reflective practice serves as a *mirror* and as a *video replay* in order to improve your professional practice.

The mirror

This image emphasises the importance of self-awareness in people-work. We need to know ourselves well enough to ensure that the particular facets of our lives enhance rather than detract from our effectiveness as workers. Some of these facets are obvious: our age, 'race', gender, how we dress, the style of language we use and our accent; these all go to make up the 'real us', and they will have an impact upon the people we work with. We always hope that such facets will not get in the way of the work we do, but sometimes they will, and we need to be aware of this.

Exercise 1

Using this metaphorical image, look at yourself in your 'mirror' and list the characteristics you observe. Have there been occasions when these have been a distinct advantage in your people-work? Have there been occasions when they have got in the way? Are you able to understand why?

Less obvious are other facets of our personality that emerge during our meetings with people, and which perhaps are drawn out of us by the other person. Our likes and dislikes, our assumptions, fears and prejudices are good examples of this. Unfortunately, if we are not aware of these, they are likely to seep out and affect our relationships with people, either through what we say, or perhaps more likely through our non-verbal communication. An honest appraisal of our true selves, 'warts and all', through this mirror of reflective practice, therefore, helps us to see where we need to be doubly careful in our dealings with others to ensure that we deliver best practice.

Video replay

In your training you may well have had the opportunity to video a simulated role-play interview to allow you to see yourself at work. There may be training opportunities in your present agency to do this. Less likely, because it is complicated by issues around confidentiality and data protection, is the opportunity to video yourself in a live interview, although in some family therapy settings this is often a useful tool.

When we talk here about video replay as a feature of reflective practice, however, we are using the term metaphorically. We are suggesting that in supervision and in training events, as well as in your own personal reflection on your practice, you 're-live' the interview, and think about the following issues:

- What went well.
- What you might have done differently.
- What opportunities you seized and those you perhaps missed.
- What feelings were stirred up in you and the other person by the content of the interview and how did you both handle these?
- How clear were your aims and objectives for the interview? Did you feel you achieved these? If so, how? If not, what got in the way?
- What issues for further reflection were brought up for you in this interview?

Note that the first question is about what went well. It is too easy to focus on the things you feel you did not do so well, but very rarely is an interview a complete disaster! Reflective practice is just as much about confirming the skills you do have and the confidence you can show, as well as exploring ways of improving your practice. Unfortunately, many people-workers, especially early on in their careers, need a lot of convincing that they can do the job well. Perhaps it is better to be like that than be over-confident, but an honest assessment of what you can do well is an important aspect of being a reflective practitioner.

A useful model

The concept of being and becoming a reflective practitioner owes much to the seminal work of Schon (1983; 1987). He used the graphic image of the 'swampy lowlands' to describe the messy business of people-work with all its problems and complications. This he contrasted with the high ground of theory and research where problems are often much more easily resolved. The skill of being a reflective practitioner, however, is to make as full use as possible of relevant theoretical perspectives and research findings in order to help those in the swampy lowlands to work towards a creative and workable set of solutions to their difficulties.

Another seminal writer was Kolb (1984), who produced a diagrammatic model about adult learning that can very usefully also be applied to reflective practice. His box diagram has four components to it, with each leading to the next. As Thompson (2002: 67) explains, these four main aspects are as follows:

Concrete experience   day to day experience forms the first step in a chain of learning.

Reflective observation   reflecting on our experience helps us begin to draw out the learning points.

Abstract conceptualisation   this stage of the learning process involved forming links between the new experience and previous learning and experience. These links build up a 'mini theory' or conceptual framework.

Active experimentation   a cycle of learning is completed when new ideas are tried out in practice.

Exercise 2

Using Kolb's model, choose an example from your own practice to see how it might work for you. If you need help, explore this with an experienced colleague, or your supervisor or practice teacher. Try it several times to get into the swing of it, and you will quickly find that this becomes something of a professional habit that develops your skills in reflective practice.

Final thoughts

There is a temptation in all people-work, especially when the sheer volume of work puts you under severe pressure, just to 'get on with it', to become almost mechanistic in your approach. The next person, just like all those who have gone before, is 'just another case', and you deal with them as best you can before moving quickly on to the next.

Perhaps what you need, as part of your commitment to best practice, is the mirror in which you creatively imagine that the next person you see could be you, or one of your children, or one of your relatives. For many workers that simple but powerful reminder is enough to rekindle their commitment to best practice, and to ensure that on a regular basis they reflect carefully on what they are doing and how they are doing it, so that everyone receives the best possible standard of help, care and support.

References and Further reading

Honey, P. and Mumford, A. (1982) *The Manual of Learning Styles*. Maidenhead: Peter Honey.

Kolb, D.A. (1984) *Experiential Learning: Experience as the Source of Learning and Development*. London: Prentice Hall.

Schon, D. (1983) *The Reflective Practitioner*. New York: Basic Books.

Schon, D. (1987) *Educating the Reflective Practitioners*. San Francisco: Jossey Bass.

Shardlow, S. and Doel, M. (1996) *Practice Learning and Teaching*. Basingstoke: Palgrave Macmillan.

Thompson, N. (2002) *People Skills*. 2nd edition. Basingstoke: Palgrave Macmillan.

Thompson, N. (2006) *Promoting Workplace Learning*. Bristol: The Policy Press.

Related concepts   Anti-discriminatory practice; establishing a professional relationship; feedback; supervision.

Religion

Some people-workers may feel surprised, shocked even, to find an entry on religion in a book devoted to communication skills. They may feel that religion is very much a private and personal matter, and that it does not have much, if any, bearing upon the work they do with people.

This view, however, needs to be challenged, and people-workers need to develop the communication skills necessary to feel comfortable about exploring religious issues, when appropriate, with people who come to them for help and support. This is not to suggest that you must become a religious expert; but it is saying that the days when anything to do with religion was regarded by people-workers as 'off the radar', have long gone. Furthermore, in the recent UK census (2001), 70 per cent revealed that they would call themselves Christian. It is also important to acknowledge that one of the motivating factors drawing some people into a people-work career is often their religious faith. Social work has its origins in religious philanthropy, and medical and nursing care also has strong roots within religious traditions.

Religion is generally regarded as a set of beliefs which are focused upon a divine power or Being, and which binds a group of believers together into a shared community relationship. It also provides a particular interpretation of how the world is to be seen and understood. Believers will share this common world-view, and often seek to persuade others of its validity. Alongside what are often referred to as 'major' religious faiths such as Christianity and Islam, for example, there is a plethora of other religious faiths and traditions which attract people's allegiance worldwide. The picture is bewilderingly complex, and it is no wonder perhaps that many people-workers do not know how to 'get started' when dealing with such matters.

Exercise 1

To help you to begin to engage with this issue, it is important to 'locate' yourself and to say where you stand on the issue of religion. For example: Are you yourself, or members of your family, religious? Can you say why this is important to you. If you are not, can you say why this is not important for you?

  This could be a lengthy exercise, of course, but it will help you explore this topic in greater depth, and its implications for your practice.

You need to think about why some people feel that religion is important. For instance:

- Some will say that their faith is central to their way of life, and provides them with a way of looking at, and understanding, the world and their place in it – in other words, their world-view.

- In our multi-faith society many people belong to a faith community where they receive, and give, support to each other in good times and bad.
- Faith communities often have a strong track record of caring for others within their local communities, including campaigning for social justice issues.
- In some areas of social work – adoption and fostering for example – Government guidelines state that workers need to be aware of, and sensitive to, the religious and spiritual needs of the children and young people whom they are placing.
- In areas of people-work such as dealing with loss, people will often ask questions about the meaning of life which may have a religious context and undertones.
- Religion for some people enables them to access power and strength to make significant changes in their lives, especially when they have been going through desperate times.
- Some researchers are publishing studies that are beginning to show a positive correlation between faith and well-being; in the field of mental health it has been claimed to play a vital part in many people's recovery.

These are some of the factors that demonstrate how religion can impact upon people as a positive influence. If this is important to the person, then it needs also to be important to the worker.

How this is conveyed, of course, is at the heart of communication skills. In the field of psychiatry, for example, Powell (2003) claims that, whereas some 80 per cent of patients felt that their religious and spiritual belief had a positive impact upon their illness, well over a third of them felt unable to discuss this with their psychiatrists. This was because they feared that their beliefs would be ignored, or seen as symptoms of their illness. These professionals were giving out a very clear signal: religion is a 'no go' area as far as treatment and well-being were concerned, and patients quickly got the message and did not raise these topics in their consultations or interviews. A similar scenario could easily be painted for other people-work professionals, including social work.

The first point to stress, therefore, is that whether you realise it or not, you will always be communicating something about your attitude towards religion when the topic crops up, even with routine form-filling. If you handle it with a tick-box mentality, you will be conveying a message that as far as you are concerned it is of little importance. If, however, you pause at that point and ask some supplementary questions, it will at least give the other person an opportunity to say whether or not this is an important issue for them. And it will have given a message that you are open to discuss it if they wish. Supplementary questions could be something like:

- How important is your religion to you?
- Do you attend a place of worship?
- Do you find your faith helps you during difficult times?

Religion can also provoke strong reactions, of course, and you need to be aware of this. In various forms it has contributed to human misery and oppression, and has been experienced by many people as a negative influence in the world. This is a view to which you may yourself strongly subscribe, and this may make it difficult for you to be open to different perceptions and experiences. But openness is a key feature of communication skills – you need to be able to put your own strongly held opinions and beliefs to one side, and to encourage the other person to explore issues that are important to them.

Even this, however, is not always easy, whether you have a religious faith or not. There are some issues on which some faith communities at least appear to subscribe to a value-base that is at odds with one which underpins all people-work. There is some antagonism, for example, in some faith perspectives towards gay and lesbian relationships, and their suitability for parenting children. The legal provision of civil partnerships is an affront to some religious people. In some faith communities the position of women is at odds with how western societies wish to celebrate equality. Jehovah's Witnesses' opposition to blood transfusions is well known, and is based upon their religious beliefs. Some workers who belong to faith communities object on principle to working with people who support abortion.

These examples have been cited because they bring to the forefront of the worker's attention some key questions which need to be asked, such as:

- Does this religious practice enrich this person's life and foster their resilience?
- Does this religious practice in any way discriminate against anyone?
- Does any of this practice seem to be abusive in any way?

If there seems to be discriminatory or abusive behaviour taking place, then clearly there is an obligation upon you to raise this, and find appropriate ways to challenge it. Certainly you will need to consult your manager for advice and guidance, but to do nothing is not an option if you suspect abuse is taking place.

Exercise 2

Spend some time with your colleagues, supervisor or practice teacher exploring some of the issues outlined in the previous paragraphs. What do you feel is the most appropriate response to make? Where do you draw the line between religious and cultural practices and abuse? Have you had any experiences within your own team where these issues have come to the fore? How were they dealt with?

Final thoughts

As in many cases of people-work, the issue of religion and religious practice throws up some key challenges to us, not least in how and what we communicate to others as representatives of our agencies. Perhaps the key questions in all such situations are these:

- To what extent does a person's religion and religious faith enrich and enhance their life, or diminish it?
- Does their religious faith strengthen or weaken their capacity and resilience to deal with life's difficulties and tragedies?
- To what extent does it give them a satisfying cohesive and enriching world-view?
- Is there any evidence that there is a risk of abuse in what they are doing as a result of their religious practices?

How we communicate with other people in this area, both verbally and non-verbally, is all important, and perhaps one of the greatest challenges to our communication skills as people-workers today.

References and Further reading

Canda, E. and Furman, L. (1997) *Spiritual Diversity in Social Work Practice: The Heart of Helping*. New York: The Free Press.

Moss, B. (2005) *Religion and Spirituality*. Lyme Regis: Russell House Publishing.

Powell, A. (2003) *Psychiatry and Spirituality: The Forgotten Dimension*. Brighton: Pavilion/NIMHE.

Royal College of Psychiatrists (2006) *Spirituality and Mental Health*. London: Royal College of Psychiatrists.

Related concepts   Anti-discriminatory practice; loss; reflective practice; spirituality.

Report Writing

(*see* court room skills)

Resilience

(*see* empowerment)

Spirituality

There is a growing interest in spirituality in contemporary society, evidenced by a burgeoning bookshop trade in alternative therapies, systems and practices of meditation, various 'new age' religions, and what seems like 1001 ways in which to find peace and fulfilment in an increasingly frenetic western society. The appeal of various eastern mystic and spiritual traditions is increasing, and many religious groups are experiencing a surge of interest as more traditional forms of religion seem to be in rapid decline.

As a concept, however, spirituality is notoriously difficult to define. People who belong to faith communities are likely to respond with definitions that reflect their religious and devotional practices, such as prayer, meditation and worship. Spirituality points them towards a deeper 'divine' mystery, a sense of awe, wonder and beauty. It also can motivate them to serve and care for others and struggle for social justice. If, by contrast, you ask someone who has no links whatsoever with a religious faith or community, they may respond by using such ideas as 'well-being', meaning and purpose, and what enriches life and makes it worth living. They too may talk about mystery, awe and wonder, but without any 'divine' or 'otherworldly' connotations. They too will seek to care for others and improve society by challenging injustice. Spirituality thus may be seen to be a 'signposting' or 'gateway' word that has a range of meanings across a wide spectrum, but which nevertheless has some common features.

The significance of all of this for our communication skills as people-workers is that we will often find ourselves engaging at quite a deep level with people, often at times of crisis and loss. Such momentous events in people's lives often evoke the unanswerable questions of 'Why': 'Why should this happen to me?'; 'Why does God allow this to happen?'; 'What have I done to deserve this?' Such inchoate and painful outpourings are not easy to respond to with integrity. It is not our role to offer 'answers', but we are sometimes called on to share the other person's distress. It is for this reason that we need to think about the communication skills that are necessary in such situations.

> **Exercise 1**
>
> Think about what we have so far raised in this discussion. Are you able to identify situations in your own life, or the lives of people with whom you have worked, where issues of spirituality have been raised or hinted at? What seemed to be the underlying issues and concerns? How were you able to respond?

The 'territory' to which spirituality points us seems to have some or all of the following features:

- people's need to feel somehow connected to something wider or 'beyond'
- a sense that something is missing in their lives: a feeling of emptiness, and being without hope or purpose in life
- a sense of not being of value – of not mattering to anyone
- feelings of being hurt, or damaged in some way
- a sense that life has let them down, and they have not got what they deserve
- feelings of guilt
- the need to make some sense of life, and to find a world-view that is sufficiently satisfying to deal with the mess, as well as the glory, of living
- questions about where people draw their strength from, especially in times of need
- questions about who or what, if anything, is 'in control'
- questions about what they are going to do with their life
- questions and worries about what happens after death.

These are some of the difficult areas of human living that prompt questions about spirituality when our often rather cosy world-view is disturbed or even shattered. *We thought we had the measure of things, but now this has happened, we are not so sure – and it hurts.*

The other side of the coin, of course, is when people's world-view proves to be sufficiently durable, flexible and resilient to absorb such painful questions and to remain intact; it then gives the person greater strength to cope even with the unanswerable nature of awful things happening.

Some guidelines to consider

When trying to deal with these issues, there are some guidelines for our communication skills that are important to grasp. These include:

- **Being, not doing** When people are feeling in touch with these profound and at times often distressing feelings, it is more helpful for you simply to be there with them. Sometimes it helps the other person just to know their space is being shared for a while, to ease their aloneness.
- **Asking, not telling** It is so tempting to offer answers to what in the end are unanswerable questions. It makes us feel better. But even if our responses satisfy us, there is no guarantee that they will satisfy the other person.
- **Going with the flow, not forcing the agenda** There will be occasions when it is more important to let the other person dictate the speed at which your interview flows, and what is discussed. Sometimes these issues may emerge in the middle of a session that you have carefully prepared and timed. Resist the temptation to get the interview back on track: you will be more helpful to them if you let them explore their difficult feelings and reactions.
- **Being humble, and not a 'know-all'** All professional people-workers are in some ways experts, and it is one of the pleasures of the job sometimes to be able to use that expertise in an effective and appropriate way. With spirituality, however, none of us is expert enough to provide answers for other people. Instead, we all have to find our way through this complicated territory. Our role as people-workers in such situations is to seek to share their journey as companionably as possible. This involves stepping back from our own expertise and being open and humble enough to let them find their own way with whatever support we are able to offer.

There are, however, some questions and comments you can pose that may prove helpful to the person going through this inner turmoil and trying to make sense of what is happening to them. These may include:

J, in what ways is all of this difficult for you to get your head around?

Does all of this make you wonder what it is all about, J?

Do you think, J, that there is someone or something who is supposed to be running the show?

Do you think that somehow it has all gone wrong?

J, do you ever try to pray when you run into difficulties?

How did you see your world, J, before all this happened? How is it different now?

Do you think, J, there is a higher power we can turn to in some ways?

How do you normally handle things when they go wrong, J?

Whom do you tend to turn to, J, when you need help and support?

Do you believe in fate, J? Do you read your horoscope? Do you believe it?

None of these questions is foolproof, of course. The most important thing is to find your own authentic style in such situations, so that you are being the 'real you'. You need to be able to communicate to the other person that you are concerned for them; that you are not going to give them a set of glib, easy answers, and that as far as you can, you are willing to share some of their journey with them. To be able to communicate those messages is the real skill: it speaks volumes about your shared humanity, and is an approach that may be far more empowering that you ever realise.

Another significant contribution to this debate has been made by Zohar and Marshall (1999), who have added the concept of Spiritual Intelligence (SQ) to the existing theoretical frameworks of IQ and Emotional Intelligence. By using this concept of SQ these writers encourage us to see a spiritual dimension in ourselves and in others, and offer some core indicators that have strong connections to people-work practice. These include:

- the capacity to be flexible
- a high degree of self-awareness
- a capacity to face and use suffering
- a capacity to face and transcend pain, and
- the quality of being inspired by vision and values.

The concept of SQ brings another strand of meaning and richness to this theme of spirituality, reminding us of the importance of taking it seriously.

Exercise 2

This discussion about spirituality has opened up a range of issues that may not regularly feature in your supervision sessions or professional discussions. In some ways they are profoundly philosophical, and demand a level of personal honesty from us in dealing with them. Whom would you feel safe to talk about such things with? What are the topics and issues that are important for you to discuss with them? Why not arrange to meet and see how you get on?

Final thoughts

One of the reasons for our own discomfort when dealing with difficult issues is that questions are raised that we may not have faced in our own lives, and therefore find extremely uncomfortable when others raise them. The temptation to run away is strong, and to allow our own discomfort to determine the agenda. There is a personal challenge in this theme of spirituality, therefore, to each one of us to try to clarify our own world-view; to test out how satisfying it is for us, and how we would cope with events that challenge its value for us. The journey of spirituality is the journey of being human, and every now and again we are privileged to share another person's painful journey in our role as people-worker. To flinch from that privilege is not only to let the other person down; in so doing we will be letting ourselves down too.

References and Further reading

Canda, E. and Furman, L. (1997) *Spiritual Diversity in Social Work Practice – The Heart of Helping*. New York: The Free Press.
Moss, B. (2005) *Religion and Spirituality*. Lyme Regis: Russell House Publishing.
Zohar, D. and Marshall, I. (1999) *SQ: Connecting with our Spiritual Intelligence*. London: Bloomsbury.

Related concepts   Anti-discriminatory practice; establishing a professional relationship; religion; reflective practice.

Strengths Perspective

(*see* empowerment, resilience and a strengths perspective)

Summarising

(*see* active listening)

Supervision

Many people-workers have mixed feelings about supervision. They agree with the rhetoric about its importance, but often report that the reality is quite different, with sessions that are more tokenistic than being really helpful to develop and sustain best practice. As Thompson (2006: 75) notes:

> Some people see it primarily or even exclusively as a means of ensuring that sufficient quality and quantity of work is being carried out – what is often referred to as 'snoopervision'.

Supervision for people-workers is nevertheless essential, because:

- It provides the structure for accountability to be maintained and exercised, as your work is scrutinised and evaluated.
- It provides an opportunity for your learning and professional development to be checked and improved so that your practice skills and knowledge continue to be honed.
- It provides opportunities for your Continuing Professional Development (CPD) to be discussed and planned.
- It provides a context in which you can be supported and encouraged.

Supervision gives expression to the central tenet of people-work, that it is a shared responsibility; you do not have to soldier on alone or in isolation. It also reinforces the basic principle that in doing your work you are a representative of the agency that employs you, and are fundamentally accountable for the work you undertake.

Exercise 1

Think about some experiences you have had of supervision. What has worked well for you? Have you had instances of poor supervision? What are the hallmarks of good supervision in your opinion? And how did poor supervision make you feel?

When thinking about supervision – whether you are offering the supervision or receiving it – it is important to recognise the centrality of good communication skills. In some ways the supervision relationship mirrors the professional relationship we seek to develop with our service users. The same skills, including verbal and non-verbal communication skills, will be in evidence, and the success of the outcome will depend in no small measure upon how well the communication between you both has taken place.

There are several books you can read to explore supervision in depth, but here are some of the key points you need to bear in mind, whether you are the supervisor or supervisee.

- Always come well prepared; know why you are meeting and the issues you need to talk about. Be open to each of you contributing to the final agenda.
- Agree the date, time and venue for the meeting and be sure to keep the appointment. If an extreme emergency crops up, consult with the supervisor in advance if possible to agree to the re-scheduling of your session.
- Decide what room layout best meets your needs.
- Ensure that you are not disturbed. Inform the receptionists that you are in supervision and for them not to put calls through to you. Switch off your mobile phone and/or pager.

All of these points help you communicate clearly that you are taking supervision seriously and want to make the very best of the time you have together.

Verbal communication skills

There is no set of specific skills for supervision; you will use the same communication skills as for everything else, but you will need to pay particular attention to what is most appropriate. For example, when discussing cases you will focus specifically on the detail and the aims and objectives of your intervention, and any feelings that have been generated which may have an impact upon your performance with that person. In the part of the meeting that deals with support, however, you will feel more able to be wide ranging in your comments and voice issues of concern, worry and debate. The extent to which this proves helpful, of course, will depend upon the relationship you have with each other professionally: the greater the trust between you, the more helpful this aspect of your discussions will be.

Specific attention should be paid, however, to the following:

- **Be assertive** You need to know what the supervision session should be achieving. If this is not happening, you need to say so, firmly but politely, and ask for specific issues to be addressed. Do not leave the session smouldering with resentment that key issues have not been tackled.

177

- **Be open and reflective** Your work involves the way in which you interact with people and how they respond to you. Supervision, therefore, will often entail some scrutiny of you as a worker, and unless you are willing to engage with that process you will not be able to improve your practice. Remember that critical appraisal of your performance is just that: a critique of your *performance*. It is not a personal attack on you as you. The best workers are always keen to learn how to improve and do better next time.
- **Be responsive** This flows from being reflective. Regard supervision as an opportunity for real dialogue. It is not a one-way process. This does not mean that you always will agree with what the other person says: a frank exchange of opposing views can become extraordinarily insightful at times. But always seek to develop the skill of showing responsiveness so that it is clear that you are committed to improving your practice. If you allow yourself to become defensive and put barriers up, then you will be letting yourself down.
- **Be accurate** Whether you are seeking to explain some aspect of your work, or are recording the notes from your supervision session afterwards, always seek to be accurate, truthful and honest. It may be difficult at times to admit to giving a poor level of service to someone, or to allowing certain feelings to cloud your judgment, but an admission and discussion of these will help to ensure that you do better next time.

A note of caution

To some of you, these guidelines may feel utopian because your experience of supervision has either been non-existent, or you have been supervised by a line manager in whom you place very little trust. Indeed, you may suspect that if you tell things 'as they really are' you may receive less rather than more support, or even be 'cold-shouldered' or punished in some way. You may even fear that promotion opportunities, and future references, may be put in jeopardy. This can be a real 'double-bind', and it would be naive to suggest that there is an easy answer.

Some suggestions are worth considering, however, to see if you can improve the quality and usefulness of your supervision sessions. For example:

- Share your concerns with another colleague whom you can trust; see if they have had similar experiences.
- Write a note to your supervisor before your next session, offering items for the agenda, specifically asking for a discussion on issues you wish to raise.

- In the session itself, take the initiative to raise such issues. You will want to choose these carefully, of course, if you are feeling uneasy about exposing your vulnerability.
- Check your job description and agency policies to see what mention is made of supervision and the expectations of supervision.
- Raise the matter tactfully in a team meeting to see if there are ways in which, as a team, supervision can be made more rewarding for everyone concerned.
- You may wish to consider raising your issues informally with a member of the senior management team to see if something can be done.
- If all of this fails, you may wish to consider using the complaints procedures so that the senior management of the agency is made aware of your concerns.
- As a last resort you need to be asking yourself if this is really the kind of agency you should be working for. Maybe the time has come to look for something better.

In all the suggested approaches outlined above, your communication skills and tactfulness will be fully tested. Think carefully about how you will broach these issues, and ensure you do it in a calm, professional manner. Keep notes of everything you do and say, and of all the responses you receive.

Exercise 2

Returning to the list you compiled in Exercise 1, think about the poor examples of supervision you listed. In light of the points raised above, how might you have tried to rectify the situation? What tactics and approaches do you think might have helped improve matters?

Group supervision

Many agencies, especially those heavily involved with training recently qualified or student workers, will make use of group supervision as part of the supervisory relationship. How this works in practice may vary depending on the supervisor. But of the four functions of supervision mentioned at the outset, only the first two are really appropriate for group supervision, namely discussion of the work being undertaken, and the teaching and development of the knowledge and skills needed for the work. Although group supervision can be enormously supportive for everyone concerned, anything that is specifically personal to an individual should not be raised in a group session, but should be kept for a one-to-one supervision session. Concern for appropriate confidentiality, in other words, should be high on the agenda.

Group discussions require a certain discipline and a willingness to follow ground rules so that everyone can contribute and benefit. The communication skills necessary for successful group supervision include:

- Don't interrupt when someone else is talking.
- Don't 'hog the show'; be brief and to the point when talking yourself.
- Be willing to take part – do not sit in silence and let all the others do the work.
- Remember that you will have useful things to contribute to help others learn, as well as gaining benefit from listening to them.
- Encourage reticent members to participate: remember that some people do find it quite difficult to speak up in front of the group.
- Don't be afraid to ask questions. It is easy to feel reticent in front of others, and to feel a little foolish asking about what you think you will be expected to know already. Remember, though, that there should be no such thing as a 'silly question', and that for everyone who asks the question there will be several more who will be grateful that you have done so.
- Keep to the agreed time for discussions, and try to keep to the point.
- Respect the group leader, who from time to time may need to move the discussion forward, even if you don't feel ready to do so.
- Find ways of ensuring that your needs are met. If for any reason you leave the meeting with unresolved issues, make a careful note of them and raise them with your supervisor next time you meet, or send a note asking for time to discuss your issues further. This is all about taking responsibility for your own learning.
- Group leaders, of course, have a specific responsibility to ensure that the group keeps to the agreed tasks, and that dominant members do not take over the discussion to the detriment of others. But it is also up to group members to be keen to contribute and to challenge anyone who is behaving inappropriately.

Final thoughts

Insisting on good supervision, whether you are the supervisor or supervisee, is part of your core commitment to best practice. It is a defined mechanism for taking good care of yourself professionally so that you can deliver a high quality service to those who come to you and your agency. Good supervision, therefore, is what you, and they, deserve.

References and Further Reading

Hawkins, P. and Shohet, R. (2000) *Supervision in the Helping Professions*. 2nd edition. Buckingham: Open University Press.
Martin, V. and Henderson, E. (2001) *Managing in Health and Social Care*. Abingdon: Routledge.
Parker, J. (2004) *Effective Practice Learning in Social Work*. Exeter: Learning Matters.
Thompson, N. (2006) *Promoting Workplace Learning*. Bristol: The Policy Press.

Related concepts Confidentiality; feedback; reflective practice.

Talks and Presentations

It is becoming increasingly important for people-workers to be able to prepare and deliver good quality talks and presentations. This is not only sometimes in your job description; it is often part of the selection process for getting the job in the first place. Good quality communication skills are essential, and some time spent on practising and improving these skills will work wonders both for your confidence and your effectiveness as a communicator.

Exercise 1

Make a list of the occasions and opportunities both within your agency and beyond, where talks and representations are needed from time to time. These can range from very low-key, informal talks involving a small number of colleagues, to more formal 'set piece' occasions.

Think of some of the talks and presentations you have attended. What marks out the good ones from the mediocre or poor ones? Note these points down and keep them to hand to refer to in the discussion that follows.

The skills you need to deliver a good talk or presentation are not in themselves difficult, but attention must be given to them if you are to succeed. When you listen to a good speaker, it all seems to be effortless, but in order to reach that standard, a lot of work has to be done by way of preparation.

There are three things you need to know: your audience and its context, your material, and your limitations.

Knowing your audience and its context

It goes without saying that knowing the nature of the audience is of vital importance. The approach you may take with a group of senior managers will be different from how you would tackle a group of interested school students wanting to know about your work. Key questions to which you need detailed answers in advance include:

- Who exactly will be there?
- What do they want to know about?
- What level of knowledge can you assume they already have?
- What is the title and topic of the talk?
- How long do they want you to talk for?
- Is there an expectation that there will be questions and discussion to follow?
- Are you the only speaker? Have others been invited to talk about other topics?
- Why precisely have they asked *you* to give the talk?
- What is the venue like? Is it a formal or informal setting?
- Who will act as convenor and chair of the meeting? Is it possible to talk to them in advance to help you in your preparation?
- What facilities are there for using visual aids, OHP acetates and/or powerpoint?
- Do they need a digest or summary in advance of the meeting?
- Is there an expectation that you will provide handouts? If so, whose responsibility will it be to ensure there are enough copies for everyone?
- What is the expected 'dress code' for the occasion?
- Are expenses or a fee paid? If you are doing this as part of your work, how will this be negotiated?
- What permissions will you need from your agency to undertake this work?
- Will you know anyone in the audience, or is it likely to be a complete 'sea of strangers'?
- How much time do you need to prepare for this event? Do you need to negotiate this with your manager?
- Is there a lectern or desk for you to put your notes on?
- How will you get feedback afterwards? Will they welcome a feedback sheet being provided for them to complete and return to you?

This may seem at first to be a bewildering set of questions and issues to tackle in advance, but if you reflect carefully on them you will begin to appreciate that the answers you receive to each of them is an important part of the preparation jigsaw. Importantly, this information will help you feel more confident and well prepared by reducing the 'areas of unknown'. The more you can feel in charge of things, the more confident you are likely to feel.

183

Know your material

You will perhaps have had some previous experience of being in a meeting with an ill-prepared speaker who mumbles, constantly shuffles through a sheaf of notes, and seems unable to communicate effectively with you as an audience. You most definitely do not want to be like that! And you won't be, *if* you follow some basic guidelines in your preparation These include:

- Survey the range of issues and information that is relevant to the subject. It is likely that you will know at least two or three times as much information as you have time to deliver. Spend time, therefore, selecting material that will be most appropriate.
- Decide what can be done within the time. Clearly, if you are giving an overview of a subject for 15 minutes, you can only briefly highlight three or four main themes. If you have an hour, then you need to decide whether to go wider or deeper. You could keep to the same three or four points and say a lot more about each one; or you could increase the themes you cover to seven or eight. In some ways, only you can decide this, but it may help to discuss the possibilities with the person who is running the meeting to see what they think would be most helpful.
- Think about how you can bring the subject to life. Are there stories you can tell which illustrate the themes you are covering? These must, of course, be totally anonymised, but the human 'slant' often helps to bring a topic to life and captures the attention of the audience.
- What visual aids will support your talk? If you are using OHP acetates or powerpoint, remember the golden rule about not putting too much information on any one slide. Ensure that your slides are clear and succinct. Think about what the audience will find most helpful.
- Having chosen your material, decide in what order you wish to present the topics you have selected, and how much time to give to each theme. Is there a particular 'take' or approach that will help the audience to remember what you are saying ? An example, or a real life (anonymised) story for instance, or some topical reference from the news or a TV series can illustrate the importance of the theme, and locate it in the minds of the audience.
- What 'props' will you need to ensure that you remember what you need to say? This will vary enormously, but most speakers need some sort of 'comfort pad' that contains their notes to which they can refer. The secret of all of this is getting the balance right between referring to notes or even the full length script, and actually talking

to the audience. The more you can maintain eye contact with the audience, the more effective you will be in your delivery. But only the most experienced can memorise what they want to say and deliver it without any notes at all. And even they can 'dry up' sometimes and find their minds go blank – so you do need to have notes easily to hand. You need to decide what will work best for you, and then to prepare fully.

- Some people like to use a set of small cards to write down the main points, to which they can refer as the talk unfolds. Whatever works for you is fine, but remember to write clearly: in the heat of the moment you need to be able to see what you have written at a glance.

- Rehearse your talk – both by yourself and with a supportive friend. This serves several purposes. It begins to give you the 'feel' of delivering the material and making it your own. You will begin to develop your own personal style and gain confidence. It will also test out the time it takes to deliver the talk. You do not want to run out of things to say with five minutes left for you to fill, or to find that you have entered 'injury time' with only a few minutes left, and you are only half-way through your material. You will be surprised in your early days of giving talks about how little, or how long, it takes to get your material over to people. Clearly, you should not rattle through the talk at breakneck speed in order to get the most information across. You will lose people in the first thirty seconds if you do that. Nor should you adopt a slow, laborious and heavy style that makes five minutes feel an eternity. Try to be your usual self with a conversational style, but vary the speed of the delivery to maintain interest. Remember that an audience's attention span can be quite limited, so break up your talk into easily identified sections and chunks.

- Practise using the OHPS or powerpoint slides and talking to them as background so that you are comfortable with the technology.

- Humour can be a good communication skill to use, but be careful. Use it sparingly, and ensure that it is appropriate to the occasion, and that you can deliver it confidently. A humorous story or joke that does down like a lead balloon is counter-productive and can be difficult to recover from.

- Think about the 'music' of your voice. Whatever the content of your talk, the delivery will be what makes or breaks it. A monotonous delivery will quickly lose the audience, for whom it will feel like a recitation from the telephone directory. By contrast, too 'sing-song' a delivery can be jarring and offputting. Try to be natural, but to use as much variation in your tone and pitch as possible.

Exercise 2

Listen to the professionals on the television or radio news bulletins. Listen not so much to what they are saying but how they say it. Close your eyes as you listen to them. Very rarely will they speak two or three words together on the same 'note' (notes, that is, as in musical notes) There will be subtle variations in order to maintain your interest. That is what you are aiming at!

Tape-record your talk – or part of it – and then listen to yourself, and see how you can improve the 'music' of your spoken delivery.

Know your limitations

Part of the confidence you will develop will rely on how well you perform on the first few talks you give. If they go well, you will feel relieved with a surge in confidence. You can get quite a buzz from a well-delivered, well-received talk or presentation. By contrast, if you have tried to be too ambitious, and have attempted to use complicated visual aids that have not worked well, you can quickly feel deflated and not want to put yourself into the 'lions den' ever again. In the early days, therefore, try not to overstretch yourself and be too ambitious. A simple, straightforward talk that is well prepared and well delivered will always go down well: someone who tries to be a 'clever clogs' is likely to lose the audience's sympathy, and they will remember only that the speaker tried to be 'too clever by half'; the content of the talk itself is likely to have been lost.

On the day itself

However well prepared you are, it is inevitable that you will feel nervous about the occasion. Believe it or not, this is to be welcomed! It means you are taking the event seriously. Anyone giving a performance, even 'old hands', will say that nervousness beforehand is an essential ingredient for ensuring that the adrenalin flows and you give of your best.

Some useful tips include the following:

- Ensure you know exactly where you have to go, and arrive in good time.
- When you arrive, look for the person in charge to let them know you are there.
- Check the layout of the room and see whether you need to make any adjustments to the furniture. You do not want to be totally hidden by a huge lectern or reading desk, or to find that there is nowhere to put your notes to enable you to refer to them easily.

- Check the equipment you will be using. If you have brought your own laptop, check that it works, and set it up in good time. If you are using their equipment, ensure that you are comfortable with how to use it. Do not be afraid to ask for help if it seems determined to thwart you!
- Check whether there is a Public Address (PA) system and whether you will need to use a microphone. If so, is this on an adjustable stand, or clipped to your lapel, or a hand-help 'lollypop'? Make yourself familiar with it, and check the voice level before the meeting so that you know how best to speak. Remember that good PA systems work best if you use your normal speaking voice, but some of the equipment you encounter may need to be tamed in advance! PA systems are also important for people who use hearing aids, so do not get into the habit of offhandedly refusing to use it or saying that you do not need it, or do not like to use it. Other people may well need it, and you must be sensitive to their needs. The hand-held 'lollypop' microphones can pose an additional hazard, of course, especially if you are using other visual aids or working your laptop. Spend a few moments getting things in the right place on the table. Maybe you will need to ask someone else to operate the laptop for you in order to have at least one hand free.
- Many people like to have a glass of water available. Do ask if one is not already available on the table for you.
- Check the order of proceedings and where you should sit before you are called to speak.
- Double check your notes and everything you need.
- If you are offering a brief feedback sheet for the audience to complete afterwards, ask the chair if you can distribute them beforehand on people's chairs. This saves you forgetting, or having to hand them out in a rush afterwards.

What to do about handouts

You will need to decide what approach to adopt about handouts, assuming of course that you have prepared one. There are two schools of thought about handouts: give them out at the beginning or give them out at the end. There are advantages (+) and pitfalls (−) with each approach and you need to decide which will work best for you.

Giving them out in advance

+ People can see the points you are making and have the overview at their fingertips.
+ They can make their own notes on the handout, especially if it adopts the powerpoint layout with space for notes against each slide.

+ You can add complex information, charts, diagrams, pictures and quotations that you can refer to during the talk, and ask people to read more easily than putting such complex information on a screen in front of them.

- People are likely to jump ahead and look for what you are going to say, rather than concentrating on the actual talk.
- People will study the handout, and you have the riveting prospect of talking to a sea of bowed heads.
- People often drop them during the talk and scrabble around noisily to retrieve them.
- Handouts invite people to use them as scribble pads for jottings, comments or games of 'noughts and crosses', which have nothing to do with your talk.

Giving them out afterwards

+ People do not have a paper-based distraction. They can focus all their attention on you and what you are saying.
+ You have some greater flexibility in how you deliver your material. If you do not stick slavishly to the order of the material as laid down in the handout, no one will know, whereas if they are following your points and you deviate from them, they will go into a mass panic and begin nervously to check with each other why there is such a major change in the proceedings.

- People do like to have the chance to make their own notes, and to jot down their questions and comments as the talk proceeds, and a handout stimulates this process.
- Some people like to use a handout to do some lateral thinking about the issues you raise, as well as paying attention to what you are saying. It is a kind of mental multi-tasking, and many people are quite good at it.

The choice is yours, and it may be a case of trial and error for the first few occasions. If you do decide to give them out at the end, then it is important to let people know this at the beginning. It saves the frantic looking for a sheet of paper, and then their scribblings as they try to keep up with what you are saying, fearful that they may lose some of the gems you are sharing with them.

Getting onto your feet

Once you are called to give the talk, there are some golden rules that will stand you in good stead, whether you have done this sort of thing many times before, or whether this is your 'baptism by fire'! These include the following:

- Stand comfortably in front of your audience, and generally keep still. A fidgety speaker, who rocks to and fro, or who makes unnecessary movements can be distracting. After you have given several talks, you will develop your own style that may involve some modest movement, but unless you do it well it can be distracting.
- Before you utter a single word, look at the audience and give them a smile. This communicates a welcoming approach from you, and immediately begins to engage your audience. You need to try to make that essential human connection between yourself and the audience from the word 'go', and a smile is a great way to begin to do that.
- It is often appropriate to begin by thanking the chair for the invitation. You may wish to add that you feel honoured and privileged to be invited.
- It is helpful to state at the outset that you have been allocated a certain amount of time to speak, and that you intend to allow some time for questions and discussion after your presentation is finished. You may want to invite people to interrupt you and ask questions as you go along, but that takes some doing! It is better for your peace of mind, at least in the early days of giving talks, to keep the questions to the end.
- Do not begin by 'running yourself down', or by apologising for your lack of experience. Of course you may feel desperately nervous, but remember that you have been invited to give this talk and that you have already given it 'your best shot' in terms of preparation. Smile, and then get on with it. The audience will come to its own conclusions about what they think of you. Be proud that you are there, and are going to do your best.
- Whether or not you have the use of a PA system, check at the outset whether you can be heard. If people ask you to speak louder, do so; but invite them to raise a hand if at any time they find you have reduced the volume.
- Remember the preparation you gave to the pace, clarity and delivery of your talk, and the 'music' of your voice. You will be surprised how easily all this goes out of your mind in the heat of the moment, and despite your best intentions you begin to gabble. Remember to take pauses, to breathe deeply, and to have short breaks in between sections. Take your cue from the audience: watch them, and that will give you a clear indication whether you have their attention or not.
- Observe the golden role of saying what you plan to say, say it, and then stop. Do not try to improvise unless you are very experienced.

Let the audience draw more out of you through their questions. This of course can be a bit daunting, but you can only do your best. It is likely that you will be so absorbed in the discussion that you will find yourself answering questions easily and in no time at all the meeting will be over. It is helpful also at the outset to give some pointers to what issues you are going to cover in the talk, and then at the very end briefly to recap before giving your final comments. This helps to clarify the structure of your talk in their minds, and acts as useful 'aide memoires' for the audience.

- If you are using OHP or powerpoint slides, try to avoid the temptation of turning to the screen behind you and talking to the slides. Keep talking to the audience; they can see the slides, and will prefer to see your face than the back of your head, especially if you are not using a PA system. Only turn to the screen if you need to point out something of key importance.
- If, during question time, you cannot answer a question, you may feel unnerved and begin to panic. Once again, the golden rule is to take your time; take a deep breath, and respond as honestly as you can. If there is nothing you can say, then it helps to reply by thanking the questioner for their comment and question, and simply say that you do not know how best to respond. Say that you would like more time to think about it, and that you would welcome an opportunity to take this matter up at a later date. The audience will usually respond sympathetically to an honest reply. After all, it is better to be upfront and say you do not know, rather than prattle on inanely for five minutes, thereby demonstrating conclusively to them that what they suspected really is true.
- At the end, thank the audience for their attention and for their invitation. It is then often custom and practice for either the chair or a designated person to offer a vote of thanks to you. Enjoy the accolade and respond with a warm smile.
- If there is facility or opportunity to obtain feedback from the audience, do make good use of it. If you have provided a simple feedback sheet, invite people to complete them and leave them in the box at the door. (You did remember to put a box by the door beforehand, didn't you?)

Tackling the gremlins

It would be wonderful to be able to say that each and every talk you give will be trouble-free, but that would be naively optimistic. Things can and do go wrong, and you will then have to think on your feet to decide how best to respond. Here are some classic examples of 'gremlins' at work:

- the powerpoint suddenly freezes on you and refuses to respond to your urgent finger-tapping pleas
- the bulb in the OHP blows and there is no spare to replace it
- in an unguarded moment you knock your glass of water all over the table and your notes – it might even spill onto the chair's lap!
- there is an unexpected fire alarm
- someone's mobile phone goes off – or worse, your own mobile begins to play that dreadful tune you have been meaning to change for weeks
- someone in the front row falls asleep and begins to snore
- people in the back row begin to chat among themselves
- someone arrives late and causes a great disturbance as they settle into their seat
- the PA system screeches unexpectedly, or picks up the conversations from the local police station
- someone is taken ill during your talk
- you drop your notes all over the floor
- you experience an unexpected attack of hiccups or coughing, or your voice strength inexplicably fades
- in the middle of the talk, you suddenly remember that you have not made arrangements for someone else to collect the children from school
- you find the lack of personal hygiene with some people sitting near you almost overpowering
- a spider, or a mouse, decides to run across the floor causing consternation to erupt
- there is a powercut and you all are thrown into darkness.

NB: In case you think these examples are from fantasy land, they have all been experienced in one form or another by the author, though thankfully not all on the same occasion.

Such gremlins will add an unwelcome piquancy to the occasion, and how you and others handle it will have to be decided upon there and then. One thing is clear: they will make the event doubly memorable! Sometimes a touch of humour will dispel the awkwardness, but use it with care.

Exercise 2

Spend some time either by yourself, or with a colleague or friend, working through the previous section about 'Tackling the gremlins'. How might you deal with each of these scenarios?

Final thoughts

Giving talks can be some of the most enjoyable and rewarding occasions for you to use and develop your communication skills. But never forget the motto: To fail to prepare is to prepare to fail.

Further Reading

Hopkins, G. (1998) *Plain English for Social Services: A Guide to Better Communication*. Lyme Regis: Russell House Publishing.
Thompson, N. (2003) *Communication and Language*. Basingstoke: Palgrave Macmillan. www.bgrg.org

---

Related concepts   Non-verbal communication.

Telephone Skills

It is difficult to imagine any form of people-work taking place without the use of the telephone. It is a major means of communication between professionals, between agencies, and between the professional worker and those with whom they are working. Given the explosion of mobile telephone provision, and its increasing sophistication, it may sound somewhat naive to suggest that people-workers need training in the professional use of this important communication tool. Surely we are all so confident with using telephones that we will adapt effortlessly to their professional usage?

The experience of student and trainee practitioners suggests otherwise. Many find themselves overawed by having to make a professional phone call; they dislike having to use the phone in front of other, more experienced colleagues, they can become 'tongue-tied', and they find it difficult to develop a professional approach. And yet a few simple guidelines are all that is needed to get people off to a good start.

Exercise 1

Spend some time ringing various organisations, firms, shops and service providers (your bank for example). Compare and contrast the ways in which these first impressions make an impact upon you. Was the welcoming message gabbled at speed, or were you able to take in what was being said? Was it pre-recorded or live? Did you have to select various options before you spoke to a real person? Did you find the message helpful or offputting? Did their voice seem flat and monotonous, or did it come across in a warm, interesting way?

Now listen to your colleagues at work – how do they come across when they answer the phone? Is there an organisational expectation of the form of words to use when you answer the phone?

What can you learn from this exercise about how you will answer the phone at work when it rings? Write down what you think sounds best, and then try it out to see how it feels.

There are some obvious differences between face-to-face interviews and telephone conversations, and we need to develop confidence to get the best out of each. We cannot usually see the face of the person at the other end of the phone – the era of the videophone as part of the professional communications kit is still some way off! So we cannot use the body language clues to help us interpret what is being said. But the tone of voice can be very revealing, and we can convey a lot through the careful development of the music of our own telephone voice. If you need any convincing of this, record yourself talking with someone sometime (with their permission) and listen to yourself. You may be surprised that your voice is not as lively as you had thought.

Exercise 2

Spend some time listening to the news on the radio. Concentrate not on what the news reader is saying, but to the music of the voice – note how the voice rises and falls, speeds up or slows down at certain points – and how rarely two or three words are spoken on the same note. These are the experts, of course, but it illustrates how you can develop important skills; of being interested in the other person and making it easier for them to speak with you by the care you take over your 'voice-music'.

Are you who you say you are?

We tend to take for granted that the person ringing us for information is who they say they are, but can we be sure? If we know them well, it is not a problem, but in professional people-work we get telephone enquiries all the time, and we have a professional responsibility to maintain confidentiality at all times. The Data Protection Act also lays a responsibility upon us to be extremely careful about what information we divulge about other people over the telephone.

Therefore, if you are not sure, ask for the name of the person who is ringing you, their location and the number for you to ring back. This gives you time to check. Often, though, it is best to ask them to put their request in writing on official notepaper so that it can be dealt with properly.

Similarly, if you are the one making the call, explain who you are and why you require the information, and invite them to ring you back, giving your number and details. Before you ring, though, ask yourself whether this is information that you could reasonably expect to be given on the phone, or whether you should put the request in writing. How soon do you need this information? This could influence how you request it.

Silence isn't always golden

In face-to-face interviews, you can often remain silent while the other person talks, because you can give encouragement to them with your facial expression, and some appropriate sounds of encouragement. On the telephone, it does not take much silence for it to become perplexing: the other person soon wonders if you are still there, or whether you have been cut off. This means that you need to be much more verbally active, simply to reassure the person that you are still there and are listening to them. This does not means you have to use a lot more words – but a more frequent use of 'mmm', 'yes', 'I see', and so on helps to oil the wheels of a non-visual conversation.

An ear for detail

How often has an inexperienced worker put the phone down and realised too late that they have not taken down some vital piece of information, even as basic as the phone number and full name of the person they were speaking to. Remember Exercise 1? It is unlikely that you will have remembered the name of the person who was introducing themselves to you – the anxiety level of the first few seconds often blocks out these key details. It is very important, therefore, before the call is finished, that you ensure that key information is exchanged, and that you log it accordingly. After all, someone else may need to follow up this information and they will need the details about whom to ring.

The dreaded answerphone

There is every chance that you will need to leave a message for someone, asking them to ring you back. Again, it is so easy not to give enough details – or to speak so quickly that the person at the other end does not stand a chance of taking down the information accurately. The golden rule is to keep it simple: speak slowly and clearly, say who you are, why you are ringing, give the day/date and time of your call, and the number for them to ring back. Depending on the circumstances, you may also wish to give a few more brief details about what it is you wish to discuss with them.

Mobile etiquette

The use of mobile phones as part of professional practice has increased enormously in recent years. There are distinct advantages to this. You can get in touch with your office when necessary, and they can update you quickly in emergencies. Your own personal safety is considerably enhanced if you have a mobile phone you can use. The more technically advanced mobiles can also enable you to access your emails, and also 'surf the net', so that you can access information for immediate use in your meeting or with your service user or enquirer. And of course the use of text messaging opens another new world of communication, although the temptation to use the texting shorthand spellings (Gd 2 C U) should be avoided in formal written communications.

But there are rules about mobile phone etiquette that are easy to overlook. You should turn them off during meetings and interviews in order to avoid disturbance and interruptions. If you are expecting an urgent call, set it to 'vibrate' and explain to the people you are with that you are expecting a call, and apologise in advance for any likely disturbance. It is unlawful to use the mobile phone while driving. And tempting though it may sometimes be, it is not professional to play games on your mobile while sitting at the back of a boring meeting.

Final thoughts

It is very easy to allow yourself to be controlled by the telephone – remember that in the end it is there to help you in your professional practice – as a servant, not as a controller. There is no such thing as a phone that cannot be switched off!

Further reading

Koprowska, J. (2005) *Communication and Interpersonal Skills in Social Work.* Exeter: Learning Matters. (pp. 57–59)
Parker, J. (2004) *Effective Practice Learning in Social Work.* Exeter: Learning Matters. (pp. 109–112)

Related concepts   Establishing a professional relationship; reflective practice.

Time Management

How we manage our time professionally communicates important messages to others about how we view them and the work we undertake. In western society at least, great store is put on punctuality: to arrive half an hour late is tantamount to insulting the person(s) waiting for you. It conveys in terms of non-verbal communication the message that they are not important enough for you to put yourself out for them and to be on time.

And yet we all know how difficult this can be at times. You may set out with every good intention of being on time for all your appointments, but people-work is a complex activity, full of the unexpected. It only takes an unexpected crisis for your schedule to be thrown into chaos. And you can become very resentful when the people you have kept waiting are angry at you for letting them down, and are not willing to accept what (to you) are compelling reasons for lateness.

There are no absolutely foolproof strategies for perfect time management, and certainly in the early days of your people-work career you will at times struggle to balance the many, sometimes conflicting demands upon your time. If only there was an easy way to learn how to prioritise!

Exercise 1

Look back over your diary for the past two weeks. How well do you feel you managed and planned your time? Were there any occasions when you were unavoidably delayed? How did you handle this? How might you deal with it differently?

Good time management comes with experience, and it is a skill we all have to develop for ourselves. There are some useful tips that will help. These include:

- Keep your appointments diary in some detail. For example, note the address and telephone number (if available) of people, meetings and visits you arrange so that they are easily to hand if you need to contact them while out of the office. A quick telephone call to say you have been delayed will help to defuse people's anxieties about why you are late, and will reassure them that you have not forgotten them.
- Allow time for travelling and breaks. If you are not sure of an area, allow enough time for getting at least a bit lost on the first time you go there. Not everyone has 'sat nav' facilities, and even the joys of 'www.multimap.com' or similar electronic direction finders cannot guarantee total success against road works, accidents and rush-hour jams. If you are planning on several visits in one day, allow time 'for you' in your schedule, for refreshments, comfort breaks and unwinding, and for making notes on each visit afterwards so that they do not all blur into one. Try not to allow yourself to be run ragged by giving yourself too ambitious a list to tackle in any one day. If your agency provides you with a laptop, you will be able to record each visit there and then, but not everyone yet has this facility provided for them.
- Know what are your best times and your worst times. If you are a morning person, for example, you will probably want to ensure that you tackle the most demanding of tasks when your energy levels are at their best, and leave the more mundane things for later in the day when you can be a bit more on 'autopilot'.
- Ensure that you plan regular events into the diary well in advance. Team meetings and supervision sessions are good examples of this, but it is also good to allocate some time each week to catch up with reading, filing and record keeping.
- Think about your annual leave entitlement and how you want to take it. Do you have free rein, or is there an agency culture about

when leave can be taken? Plan ahead so that you have the breaks you need and deserve to avoid burn out.

- When you arrange home visits, think about what else you have to do that day, and in your appointment letter, or when you speak face-to-face, give the time you hope to arrive, and say that you will make every effort to be punctual, but explain that there may be occasions where something unavoidable crops up and you may be delayed. Forewarned is forearmed!

- Ensure that really important events, like attendance at court, case conferences, key meetings are put into your diary as soon as you know them.

- If you keep a social diary as well as a work-based diary, you need to be doubly vigilant. If you fail to take into account an important birthday, anniversary or social function, and plan to work late that evening, you will find your popularity ratings plummeting with certain people close to you. For this reason, many people keep a basic note of personal matters in their work diary to avoid such clashes. Again, to miss these events when you could reasonably have planned not to, is to communicate something about your priorities to the other person(s) involved. And there is life outside work – or there ought to be – to keep you lively and vibrant as a person. Electronic diaries, of course, present added complications if others can make appointments on your behalf. It is important, therefore, to ensure that you keep control, by making it clear when you are, and are not, available.

A note of caution

Diaries contain information both about you and those with whom you are working and visiting. You need to make reasonable steps to ensure that confidentiality is maintained in your diary. But most of all you need to keep it very safe. A lost diary is a multi-dimensional disaster to be avoided at all costs. So do keep it secure, and don't leave it unattended in the car or anywhere else.

A useful tip

It is a good idea, notwithstanding the advice given above, to photocopy your diary every now and then so that a spare copy of your appointments is available in the event of your diary going AWOL for some reason. In moments of stress we can all do things we regret, and a mislaid diary can cause all manner of complications. A photocopy kept in a safe place can really save the day.

Exercise 2

Photocopy your work diary, including the list of useful addresses and contact details that you may have compiled over a period of time, and put it in a safe place. Make a diary note at the end of the period you have copied to do it again for the next block of time so that you get into the habit.

Final thoughts

Although time is a very measured, and measurable, phenomenon, it is also a social and an emotional construct. To be late in some cultures is almost to insult people, whereas in other settings the concept of being 'late' hardly seems to occur to people. In our own lives, time can drag, stand still or fly by. And of course for some professional people, time is money! Time therefore is a multi-layered phenomenon, and in our professional lives we need to be aware of its many complexities, as well as ensuring that we make the best use of it in our work.

Further reading

Thompson, N. (2002) *People Skills*. 2nd edition. Basingstoke: Palgrave Macmillan.
Thompson, N. (2006) *Promoting Workplace Learning*. Bristol: The Policy Press.

Related concepts   Endings; establishing a professional relationship; reflective practice.

Transference

(*see* establishing a professional relationship)

Whistle Blowing

'Whistle blowing' is the term used when a worker reports another worker's serious bad practice to the management of the agency. To be in this position is perhaps one of the most difficult, and at times lonely and potentially isolating experiences you can encounter. The temptation to keep quiet and to hope that it will go away can be immense; the decision to challenge and/or report your concerns can sometimes require immense courage. And it goes without saying that the communication skills required are of the highest order for this to be done effectively.

If you have completed this exercise thoughtfully, you will have already realised how complex and potentially 'scary' this situation can be. Perhaps too you will have realised that whistle blowing is a tactic of the last resort: crucially important, but nonetheless not to be considered as the first step to take.

If you find yourself in this sort of situation – let's say, by way of illustration, that a colleague is misappropriating agency funds, or acting abusively towards a service user – you need to think carefully about what to do. The following checklist will help you clarify your thinking.

1 Are you certain about this? Is it merely a suspicion, or do you have hard evidence? If you are going to make an allegation about a colleague, you must be very sure of your facts. Imagine how you would

feel if someone 'got hold of the wrong end of the stick' and accused you unfairly of a misdemeanour.

2   Check your agency policy manual to see, first of all, whether there is a whistle blowing policy. More and more agencies are required to have one, and various training and education courses – social work for example – are required to have a whistle blowing policy in place so that students and workers are clear about such matters.

- If you do have a policy, read it through carefully: it should give you a step by step procedure to follow. It should also reassure you that it is illegal for you to be victimised in any way as a result of your report, irrespective of the eventual outcome. Things may be uncomfortable for a while, but you should not be in any way penalised.

- If you cannot find a policy in the manual, try to find out whether it is kept somewhere else. Try to ask around. This may feel difficult, of course, as people will immediately begin to wonder why you are asking! You will have to decide how to approach this. Sometimes you can explain that you are doing a comparative study or research project on whistle blowing as part of a course you are on, or out of general interest. It is always a good idea to look at other agencies' policies anyway. If you draw a blank, especially if you feel uncomfortable about probing further, then seek advice. To whom you turn will depend very much upon your status within the agency. If you are a student, for example, you should always talk first to your supervisor or practice teacher and/or your academic tutor. If, however, you are a worker in the agency, you may feel it will help to talk to an independent body for advice and information such as your local Citizens Advice Bureau (CAB). This process of fact-finding is important as it will help you decide the best course of action.

3   Seek an ally whom you can trust, with whom you can discuss things confidentially and seek support. This can be a very worrying and stressful situation to be in, and having a good supporter can sometimes make all the difference if the going gets tough.

4   Decide whether you can approach the person directly in some way. This is not easy, but it is worth considering at the outset. If you can find a quiet moment, you could tell the other person that you hope you are wrong, but that you have noticed what seems to be going on, and that this will put you in a difficult position if it continues. It is probably not wise to enter into a detailed discussion, but it will be instructive to hear the response that your statement elicits. If it is true, the other person will have been warned, and will have to do something to put the situation right.

5   If this course of action is not possible for whatever reason, then the time has come to talk to someone in authority – your supervisor or immediate line manager. They should be able to advise you about what to do next. They may tell you that they will take the responsibility to follow up your concerns and allegations without bringing your name into it, and to see that matters are properly dealt with. Unless there are compelling reasons to doubt what is being said to you, you should let the manager take it forward, and try to let the matter rest at that point. But do make a note of what you have done and said for your own records, and keep it in a safe place.

6   If all else fails, then you need to activate the formal whistle blowing procedure by writing to the senior manager or Chief Executive Officer (CEO), outlining your concerns and allegations and citing relevant evidence in support of them. Mark the letter 'strictly private and confidential' and keep a copy for your own records. Do not send it electronically – it is not always possible to guarantee that it will remain confidential or be seen only by the person to whom you have sent it. If the CEO needs to copy it to key people, that will be his or her responsibility.

7   How the agency deals with this may vary. Best practice suggests that you should be called to a meeting to discuss your allegations with the CEO in confidence, but sometimes all you may receive is a brief letter of acknowledgement. Occasionally you may not even receive that, and you may be left wondering what is happening. But you will have discharged your responsibility by sending it.

8   Always bear in mind that the best agencies will welcome whistle blowing and will want to make the process as straightforward as possible in order to maintain their reputation for high standards. Indeed, anything which undermines that, or goes against the grain of the agency's value-base deserves to be challenged, and should be welcomed. They should have the self-same set of concerns and value-base that caused you to be concerned in the first place.

Final thoughts

However much you may agree in your head with what has been said about whistle blowing, when it becomes real for you, your heart and gut may well tell another story. You may find, for example, that the aftershock may be more painful for you than you had expected; you may be made to feel very uncomfortable, victimised even. If this happens, always keep a careful note of what is happening, and if necessary lodge a complaint or a grievance. Seek legal advice, and if necessary look for another job which better reflects your own values. This is not necessarily going to be easy, but matters of deep principle and conscience are of such importance that you will know deep down that you have to do what is right if you are going to be able to continue living with yourself. It will be this sense of doing what you know to be right that will sustain you in the darker times.

Further reading

Parker, J. (2004) *Effective Practice Learning in Social Work*. Exeter: Learning Matters.
www.bvs.co.uk
www.pcaw.co.uk

Related concepts   Establishing a professional relationship; reflective practice; supervision.

'Wicked' Skills

Although to the purist any use of the term 'wicked' apart from being a synonym for 'evil' is likely to be deplored, it has now entered social care vocabulary with a different meaning, as well as being used in popular youth culture as an expression of approbation. The praise, or blame, for this development belongs to Clarke and Stewart who famously talk about wicked issues and wicked problems as being:

> Those issues for which there is no obvious or easily found solutions. They seem intractable ... there can be hope that wicked problems will be solved over time, but that requires learning ... the nature of the problems and ... their causes. They require a capacity to derive and design new approaches for their resolution, and to learn of their impact. They are likely to be resolved not directly but through an iterative process – learning, trying and learning'. (Clark and Stewart, 2003, cited in Thompson, 2006: 26)

The Open University has also done some important work on 'wicked competence assessment' through its Practice Based Professional Learning Centre.

Wicked problems require wicked skills to tackle them, skills that are involved with reflective practice and a capacity to think 'outside the box' in a creative way, by adopting what the authors call 'holistic not partial or linear thinking ... [and a] willingness to entertain the unconventional and pursue the radical (Clark and Stewart, 2003: 275).

'Wicked' in the context of communication skills also is being used to refer to a range of 'wicked competences' that are by definition hard to assess, but are also high on the list of employers' requirements of their people-working staff. Such competences include:

- developing supportive relationships
- group work effectiveness
- active listening skills
- relating to others
- self-management, including self-confidence
- emotional intelligence (EQ).

Such essential 'wicked' skills are difficult to define, and certainly not easy to assess; they are referred to sometimes as 'fuzzy' for this very reason. But of their importance there can be no doubt.

Final thoughts

Whether this concept of 'wicked' stands the test of time is open to debate, but if it provides a somewhat light-hearted approach and introduction to some serious issues, it will have served its purpose well enough. We might then go so far as to express our approval 'wicked!'

References and Further reading

Clarke, M. and Stewart, J. (2003) 'Handling the wicked issues', in Reynolds, J., Henderson, J., Seden, J., Charlesworth, J. and Bullman, A. (eds) (2003) *The Managing Care Reader*. London: Routledge.

Thompson, N. (2006) *People Problems*. Basingstoke: Palgrave Macmillan.

Related concepts Active listening; assessment; reflective practice; supervision.

Wrong Messages

The discussion about non-verbal communication skills emphasises how important it is to be aware of 'wrong' messages we can convey to people sometimes without being aware of it. Turning up late to see people can give them the impression that they are not very important and that we do not care very much about them.

More serious, however, is the possibility of giving wrong messages to the people with whom we work. This is often about workers not maintaining appropriate professional boundaries in their relationships with people.

For example, being friendly towards those with whom we work is an important aspect of establishing a professional relationship, within which we can do some important work with people. It is an aspect of empathy. But we are not actually becoming friends with the other person. Our relationship is established for a specific purpose that, once accomplished, means that the relationship comes to an end – or as we say, *job done.* It would be wholly inappropriate to keep in touch with the person, or to have coffee with them or go on a day out with them, because this would take the relationship into a more personal rather than professional sphere.

It has to be admitted that this boundary is not always easy to maintain. In some aspects of people-work it is often helpful to meet the person on what may be called neutral territory; in other words not at your office or in their home. Working with disadvantaged young people, for example, may sometimes be far more effective if the worker sees them in town, in a coffee bar or internet cafe. It conveys an important message about meeting people in territory which they feel comfortable in. But the relationship still must remain professional.

The difficulties arise because as human beings we have feelings, and sometimes deep attraction to each other. A person who has been going through emotional turmoil may feel hugely grateful to the worker for their time and concern, and for the friendly, caring approach they have adopted. They may feel that this worker has made all the difference to their lives, and a deep sense of gratitude can begin to form. They may want to show this gratitude through physical affection to the worker. And because feelings can be two-way, the worker themselves may begin to experience strong feelings about the other person, beginning first from a sense of protection perhaps, or wanting them to recover from whatever is afflicting them; but this can then move on towards a feeling of physical attraction. The service user may feel they are falling

205

in love with their worker: their feelings may be reciprocated, and a sexual relationship may then follow.

It must be said categorically that this is both unprofessional and unacceptable behaviour that flouts professional codes of conduct. Cases of this nature almost always result in disciplinary proceedings being taken against the worker, who will be deemed to have breached their position of trust, and to have exploited someone who was feeling vulnerable.

But we live in the real world of flesh, blood and lust, and it would be naive to pretend that in our professional relationships we do not from time to time find the person we are working with hugely attractive physically. It is important, therefore, that the worker takes steps not only to protect themselves against any accusation of inappropriate conduct, but also guards against entering into physical and sexual relationships. Partnership-working does not mean you can become partners!

In guarding against the over-stepping of boundaries with service users there are several important points to bear in mind. These include the following:

- Always ensure that the place and time where you meet is appropriate.
- If need be, ensure that you are not working alone with the other person.
- If feelings of attraction to a service user begin to occur, raise the issue with your practice teacher, supervisor or manager at an early stage so that you can discuss how best to deal with it.
- Be reflective: what are these feelings within you telling you about yourself, your level of self-awareness, your need to be loved and to be seen to be attractive, and your own personal relationships?
- Ensure that the non-verbal communications between you and the other person are kept within the boundaries of the professional relationship. Do not underestimate the impact of a warm look, a deep smile, or a physical touch: to someone who is feeling unloved, vulnerable and uncared for, it may be easy to misunderstand what is being communicated.
- If you sense that the other person is becoming too interested in you 'as you', remind them about the professional nature of the relationship, and always end the interview in a low-key, businesslike manner. You may even wish to use their formal title rather than their first names when saying goodbye, just to reinforce this message.

There are some other strategies that some people-workers choose to adopt, such as the wearing of a ring on their wedding finger, irrespective of whether they are in a committed relationship. Some workers – both male and female – feel that this is an important reinforcement of their professional boundaries. There will, of course, be others who fiercely eschew such a practice as being wholly dishonest, regarding it as a 'game' that they do not wish to play.

Exercise 1

Think carefully about some of the work you have done with people where you felt a degree of physical attraction towards them. How did you handle this? Are there some situations in which you feel personally that you would be more vulnerable than others? How will you plan to deal with such scenarios?

Final thoughts

It is important to reinforce the principal issue in all of this: we enter into professional relationships with people for a distinct and clearly negotiated purpose, which has an end in sight. Best practice will never lose sight of the endings from the very beginning, and will always seek to be evaluating and assessing the progress being made towards achieving the agreed objectives. The quality of the empathic professional relationship that we establish will be crucial to achieving these objectives, but once that relationship becomes an end in itself, we will have crossed a vital boundary.

Related concepts Barrier gestures; non-verbal communication; empathy; endings; supervision.

Index